PRAISE FOR

*Bless the Birds*

"*Bless the Birds* is the book for our times. It's a splendid blend of landscapes, relationships, creative work, and spirituality—finding meaning in life framed by an awareness of death. I have a dozen people I want to share this authentic, honest, hopeful memoir with—and you will, too. It's a treasure."

—Jane Kirkpatrick, *New York Times* best-selling author of
*Something Worth Doing*

"It's such a ripe time for this book about how to meet fear, loss, and sorrow with courage, grace, and most importantly, love."

—Rosemerry Wahtola Trommer, author of *Hush*

"*Bless the Birds* is spare and precise, and full of love and resilience. It's the story of two lovers taking a journey that none of us want to take: a journey toward parting. They walk it with eyes and hearts wide open, finding joy in their moments and showing just how much tenderness and grace are possible at life's endings—so much love that the reader's heart spills over with it just by accompanying them."

—Priscilla Stuckey, author of *Tamed By a Bear*

"*Bless the Birds* reminds us that dying is entwined with living, and we can do both with our hearts outstretched. Tweit shares the deeply personal story of the path she and her late husband walked, illuminating the fear, hope, bewilderment, rage, astonishment, laughter, exhaustion, gratitude, and joy when we open ourselves to life and death and love. This book is a gift for medical, palliative care, and hospice professionals as well as people navigating illness in their own lives."

—Elizabeth Holman, PhD, palliative care psychologist

# Bless
# the Birds

# Bless the Birds

## Living with Love in a Time of Dying

Susan J. Tweit

swp

Published 2021
Printed in the United States of America
Print ISBN: 978-1-64742-036-9
E-ISBN: 978-1-64742-037-6
Library of Congress Control Number: 2020917545

For information, address:
She Writes Press
1569 Solano Ave #546
Berkeley, CA 94707

She Writes Press is a division of SparkPoint Studio, LLC.

*Book design by Stacey Aaronson*

FOR RICHARD AND MOLLY—

ALWAYS IN MY HEART

*I am not saying we should love death, but rather that we should love
life so generously, without picking and choosing, that we
automatically include it (life's other half) in our love.*
—Letter from Rainer Maria Rilke to
Countess Margot Sizzo-Noris-Crouy, 1923

*I am now face to face with dying, but I am not finished with living.*
—Oliver Sacks, *Gratitude*

# author's note

This book is a memoir, meaning it is my story, mined from my recollections, supported by data from journals, blog posts, and medical records. I've done my best to be accurate and to portray the people and events involved truthfully. I recognize "truth" is a slippery concept, given that our brains revise our memories to suit our internal narratives. Hence this caveat: This is my take; others may remember these events differently.

Parts of this book appeared in different forms in the *Denver Post*, *Western Friend*, and *High Country News*, and on my blog. Much appreciation to editors Barbara Ellis at the *Post* and Betsy Marston at *High Country News*.

# introduction

*I pray to the birds because they remind me of what I love
rather than what I fear. And at the end of my prayers, they
teach me how to listen.*

—TERRY TEMPEST WILLIAMS,
*Refuge: An Unnatural History of Family and Place*

T his story is about living in a time of dying. It is both prayer
and love song, an invitation to walk in the light of what we
love, especially when times are hard or heartbreaking. To open our
hearts and go forward with as much grace as we can through life's
changes. To honor our cell-deep connection to all of the other lives
with whom we share this planet. To celebrate the miracle of simply
being, our capacity for love, which is both gift and salvation.

The "time of dying" is both personal and political. The personal is this: In 2011, I took care of both my mother and my husband through their deaths.

My mother was three months shy of eighty years old. Her
death was in the statistical norm for her race (white), class
(middle), and generation (she was born in 1931), though it was hastened by debilitating rheumatoid arthritis and the onset of
Alzheimer's disease. Norms or not, she was my mom, my fiercest
defender and most thoughtful critic. I wasn't ready.

The death of my husband, companion, partner, and lover since graduate school was unthinkable. Richard had always been robustly healthy, something he took for granted until one morning when he saw thousands of birds—the first sign, at age fifty-nine, of the brain cancer that would kill him. We journeyed with that illness for two and a quarter years, at first in the belief that his health, strength, and brilliant mind would carry him through. Finally, knowing they wouldn't, we chose to celebrate the end of our "together" by setting out on a literal journey, a three week road trip on the Pacific Coast. Along the way, I learned to be truly alive: to be present even in the worst moments, and to laugh, love, shout, and cry fearlessly. That learning is what we all need to thrive when our days turn dark.

The political is this: the times we live in. It seems that all we value—civility, respect, truth, our trust in our institutions and our own safety, the interwoven community of life on Earth—is dying. Or at least changing so radically that we no longer recognize what we once knew.

The personal is political. That feminist slogan of the 1970s reflects the truth that how we live our lives, our daily actions and interactions, are what shape culture and society. Who we are, how we treat others, what we buy, and how we spend our time—all of these become the political, a word that has its roots in *politis*, Greek for "citizen." That's us.

As a scientist trained in plant ecology, I have learned much from the photosynthesizing communities that green and shape Earth, cooperating as they breathe in the carbon dioxide that we and our carbon-consuming lives exhale, and breathing out the oxygen that sustains us. Plants are my teachers, the wild world my solace and inspiration. As climate change accelerates, I grieve for this unique planet, the only home our species has ever known. Past extinction events show that life will reemerge—if not in the form we most prefer. As Rebecca Solnit writes in "A Letter to a Young Climate Activist on the First Day of the New Decade": "The natural world is strong and resilient. This does not mean that everything is fine. It does mean that given half a chance some of the natural world will survive, and giving that chance depends on us."

That's where this story comes in. As part of giving life that chance, we humans need to let go of our phobias about death and learn to accept "life's other half." To go into our endings mindfully, with a lot less angst and wasted energy, and a lot more love and grace—especially we baby boomers, now coming into our home stretch.

Natural death is an integral part of existence. It opens space for new life; it recycles the cells, molecules, and atoms that were "us" into new forms; it keeps the larger cycle of life continuing.

Accepting death is a form of adaptation, a flexing with change, rather than fighting it. Change is one of the few constants in life, as we learned from the COVID-19 pandemic and the tumult as the United States finally began confronting its ingrained racism. The world I grew up in is not the world my stepdaughter grew up in, or the world as it will be when her kids and grandkids grow up. My hope is that we will move forward in positive ways to slow climate change, grow a more sustainable economy, and work toward a more equitable society. Whatever we do, we need to remember that change is natural, as is our profound discomfort at having to adapt, and our grief at the losses we experience along the way.

I offer this personal story as an example of something positive we can do: live with love for all, and "lean in" to nature, the community that birthed our species. I see love as humans' greatest gift to this earth, and one we need to cultivate—especially now, when racism and other toxic "isms" make life painful and perilous for those we label "other," and exacerbate the deep divisions in our country. I am white, middle-class, female, and growing old. I have lived through loss, fear, and pain. I am still walking forward, still finding joy in the lives around me, human and moreso. Still loving. I bless the birds because the sudden and profoundly unnerving appearance of Richard's avian hallucinations afforded us time to learn how to walk his journey with love. To be reminded of the kindness and generosity intrinsic in humanity. To take heart and sustenance from the miracle of life on this glorious planet, challenges and all. To live fully in a time when life seems especially hard and heartbreaking.

# chapter one

∽

## Day One

### Odometer Reading: 182 Miles

Richard opened his eyes as I slowed the car for the turn to the gravel ranch road. I lowered the windows, letting in the rich smell of new-mown hay, along with a distinctive, throbbing call: *Khrrr, khrrr, khrrr!*

"Sandhill cranes!" A smile creased Richard's tanned face. He reached for my hand. "I'm a lucky guy."

The man sitting in the passenger seat next to me had "moon face," the high cheekbones and chiseled profile gifted by a Cherokee-Chickasaw ancestor now rounded and puffy, a symptom of the steroids that controlled swelling from a growing brain tumor. His deep-set hazel eyes protruded; his muscly chest was soft. But when I looked at him, I saw only the mile-wide smile, joyous and tinged with mischief—the same smile that had captivated me when we met, almost twenty-nine years earlier; the smile that lit up everyone and everything around him. I felt a rush of love, a flood of oxytocin, that excited and terrified me as much as it did when I first became his lover. Now, I was his caregiver. He had terminal brain cancer. And we were setting off on a four-thousand-mile, belated honeymoon journey because our time together was short. Because we were determined to *live* every moment.

Scanning Richard's face, I was searching for grace, which to me is the ability to embrace life with a combination of balance, harmony, and beauty. The ability to be present, heart open, even in—especially in—the moments when our hearts want to flinch, freeze, or turn away. When all seems lost: the wounded bird dies in our hands; the strayed child is not found safe and sound; the light of life on this animate planet flickers, as if to fade out.

I swiped at tears with the hand that should have been holding the steering wheel and drove on toward the ranch headquarters, a cluster of white-painted wooden buildings. I parked in our usual spot under the spruce tree by the bunkhouse. "I'm going to haul our stuff upstairs."

"I can help." Richard pulled his six-foot length slowly out of the car and then reached behind the seat for his briefcase. I grabbed our duffel, the box with his medications, my briefcase, and his pillow. We walked across the lawn and into the historic ranch house. As I turned to go up the narrow stairs to the bedrooms, Richard stopped. "You go first," he said. *Uh-oh.*

"Richard can manage the stairs, can't he?" Betsy, the facilities manager at Carpenter Ranch, had asked when I called about our stay. I relayed the question to him.

"Of course." His voice carried the confidence of sixty-one years of having inhabited a muscular and appealingly male form. The voice of a man who could free-climb a cliff, sculpt a one-ton boulder, or juggle three balls while balancing on one leg. A man who could bound up that steep flight of steps, carrying our mound of gear. His sense of self hadn't changed, but his abilities had.

This Richard froze at the bottom step, his tumor-impaired

right brain struggling to make sense of how to ascend. I stopped at the top, arms loaded, watching with a stomach-churning mix of horror and fascination, compelled to witness the effects of the disease I could not stop. Finally, he reached for the handrail and took the steps slowly, one at a time, like an old man.

When I was a child, I knew love when Mom reached for my hand to help me up a steep bit of trail, or when Dad carried my knapsack once I tired. When my brother Bill, two years older and more popular than I, let me tag along. Love showed in my granddad Milner's quirked eyebrow and dry banter when I challenged him at chess, and when he never let me win. I understood love as a partnership based on deep respect and affection. Now, love meant fearlessly supporting my partner, the strong guy who still held my heart in his shaky hands.

We had begun visiting Carpenter Ranch, a working ranch owned by the Nature Conservancy, the previous summer, after being awarded a service residency inspired by our concept of terraphilia, humans' innate affiliation with the earth and its web of life. As Richard's website explained it, "'Terraphilia' is a word my wife and I started using to convey the notion that each of us is inextricably connected to the whole world, and that a happy, well-adjusted human being ought to have kind, loving feelings extending beyond the illusory boundaries of our skin, and we ought to recognize and acknowledge those feelings."

Our assignment: transform a half acre of unwanted, water-hungry lawn behind the ranch house into a public interpretive space that would honor the ranch and surrounding wild country. We envisioned a part-wild, part-domestic garden with sculptural structures that would, in the words of ethnobotanist Gary Paul Nabhan, "re-story" the weedy ground. An artistic landscape that would reestablish the bond between land and community. The project was our first public collaboration, melding Richard's heart work of abstract sculpture using local rocks and found industrial materials with my passion for plants as pioneers of natural restoration. We knew when we accepted the residency that Richard had brain tumors. He was healthy then, his prognosis good. We didn't imagine his life would end before the work did.

"Why didn't we do this sooner?" Richard asked, as we strolled hand in hand out the ranch driveway that evening, his stride sure again on level ground.

"The honeymoon road trip?" I asked. "Or the collaboration?"

"Both," he said, and swung our joined hands high in a joyous arc.

"We were too focused on earning a living." I kept my voice dry.

"Oh, that," said the guy with the PhD in economics. "It's only money." He grinned. "Just money!"

He chuckled over his joke until we stopped to admire the sunset flaming the western sky. Then he drew me against him, my back fitting his chest, his chin resting atop my head. "The hardest thing for me now is that I can't do much. I don't have the energy."

I chose my words carefully. "I don't think it's about the doing, sweetie. I think what matters in life is being. Your evident love for life, even now, inspires us all."

He smiled, teeth white against cherrywood-colored skin, and repeated, "I'm a lucky guy."

I gripped his hand, willing away tears. "I love you."

This wasn't our plan.

We hadn't even reached retirement, which for us, an economist turned sculptor and a freelance writer, didn't mean quitting work. It meant quitting worrying about earning money and focusing instead on work that fed our spirits. Richard had only begun to explore his art, his notebooks full of sketches and ideas about how to give native rocks their voices as "ambassadors of the earth." I found myself increasingly drawn to the service of restoring our planet, nurturing Earth's community of diverse life and lives.

When we met in graduate school at the University of Wyoming nearly three decades before, Richard was the brilliant PhD student with the soul of an artist, the one who could grasp a complex mathematical model as effortlessly as he could hike up a mountainside, move a refrigerator, or heft Molly, his cute-as-a-bug daughter, onto his shoulders. The tall and handsome guy with a dream of a college teaching post in some small town where he could buy land and build a passive solar house with his own hands, milling the lumber from trees he logged. And grow a self-sufficient, light-on-the-land existence with intellectual pursuits balanced by physical work. A mash-up of Henry David Thoreau's Walden Pond with Helen and Scott Nearing's *The Good Life*, informed by the ingenuity of the *Whole Earth Catalog*.

I was the shy, slender, and freckled field ecologist born to a family of nature-loving scientists and artists. A recent diagnosis with lupus, a potentially fatal, incurable illness, had imploded my first marriage and torched my field science career. I found refuge in a communal household practicing urban farming, with chickens and a huge garden, and graduate studies melding right-brain writing with left-brain science. I worked as the director of the campus women's center.

One of my volunteers, an econ grad student with Richard, decided that he and I would be the perfect pair. I fended off Sue's matchmaking with some crankiness. I needed a man right then "like a fish needs a bicycle," as the poster on my office wall said. Illness had unglued my old life, and I hadn't put the pieces back together yet. I was still trying to figure out the damn pattern.

Undeterred, Sue connived a meeting at her birthday that December. True to form for someone intent on cramming more into every moment of each day, I arrived late. I dashed into the restaurant and paused to wipe glasses fogged by the sudden warmth. Sue, with her patrician face and straight brown hair, waved from a long table across the crowded room.

I saw with a sinking heart that the last seat remaining was between two guys, both single dads, whom I knew only from her descriptions. One was Richard, with Molly playing at his feet.

I swallowed nervousness, sat down, and introduced myself. I know I spoke to the other grad student, but I can't recall his face. It was Richard who made my belly flutter, my breath catch, and the heartbeat rendered chronically erratic by my illness actually stumble. It wasn't so much his looks, though I appreciated his muscled form, skin sun-warmed even in the darkness of a Laramie winter, and his El Greco oval face, deep eyes, and silky black beard and mustache. It was the way those eyes held mine, his slow and beautiful smile, his musical-tenor voice, and that he listened when I spoke. As if I already mattered to him.

And three-year-old Molly in her purple corduroy overalls, with that same hair and engaging smile, who climbed into my lap and sat trustingly, eating bites of my food.

At the end of the evening, I hugged Molly, set her down carefully, and shook Richard's hand. I pulled mittens over fingers that still tingled, zipped up my jacket, and walked away. I reminded myself firmly that a man and a kid, no matter how appealing the package, were not what I needed. I had to figure out *me* first. It was winter break: I would head south to visit my parents in Arizona, and get over this flutter before I returned.

I never got over the flutter. I'm a scientist—I don't believe in love at first sight. Show me the data, not the flutter. The data are that we moved in together five weeks after Sue's birthday party and married eight months later, Molly in attendance, a crown of garden flowers in her hair.

We had a plan: create our personal Good Life with the sun-filled house in the woods and the big garden for growing healthy food. The first hitch was where.

"Could you be happy away from Wyoming?" Richard asked one evening as we walked together, Molly perched on his broad shoulders.

"I love you," I said, as two pairs of gold-flecked brown eyes watched me. "I can try."

And try I did, as Richard's career bounced us from Wyoming to West Virginia for just two semesters, and then to Washington state, where we bought land with a tumble-down farm-house we put a lot of love into. We then moved to Colorado for a year, while Richard finished his PhD and I wrote my first book, a journal of nature in town, after which Richard was offered a research post in Iowa, and off we trucked to the Great Plains.

Then came southern New Mexico's Chihuahuan Desert,

where Richard got tenure at New Mexico State University, I wrote five books about the desert, and Molly took up flute and won a music scholarship. After one "practice" semester at the university where her daddy taught, Molly, now tall, with her father's elegant bones and restless mind, left us for Portland and Reed College.

We left too, still pursuing our dream of a sustainable life. That took us north to Salida, the small town in rural southern Colorado where Richard had lived as a child. The high-desert valley bounded by the tallest reach of the Rocky Mountains didn't offer a university for Richard to teach at, but it did provide stunning scenery, friendly people, and reasonably priced land.

Within months of our move, we bought a half block of junk-strewn former industrial property. Our "decaying industrial empire," as we dubbed it, boasted a glorious view of the peaks, a dilapidated but spacious century-old brick building perfect for Richard's studio, plus space to build the passive-solar house he had envisioned for so long. It also came with frontage on a block of channelized and trash-filled urban creek, fulfilling my lifelong dream of having a creek to play with. Whenever we had both money and time, we worked on restoration. Richard began with the shop, progressing upward from the cracked concrete floor to the leaking tin roof. I weeded and planted, patiently working on healing land and creek. We were both putting down roots.

It was not smooth going. The consulting work that had allowed Richard to leave his academic post dried up, taking his income with it. His identity as a breadwinner gone, he sank into a black hole. Eventually, my patience ran out.

"Goddamn it!" I shouted one night, as he silently ate his way through the dinner I had carefully prepared. "We have savings; I have writing income. Quit feeling sorry for yourself! This is your chance to build the house you've been dreaming of. You've got a brain and muscles. Use them!"

He finished eating, stormed out without a word, and sulked in his studio for days. Then one evening, he came in with sketches of kitchen cabinets. "What do you think of ash face frames pegged with mesquite at the corners, Craftsman-style?" he asked, as if neither fight nor sulk had ever been. After that, he picked up his tools and went to work.

The next year we took on parent care, moving my folks from Tucson to Denver so we could watch over them. Two years later, we commuted the thousand-mile-drive to Arkansas each month to help with Richard's father's hospice care. The following year, Molly was diagnosed with thyroid cancer and we drove to Portland to help her weather surgery and radiation.

It's a wonder we survived, much less continued to love each other.

The July that Richard turned fifty-six, the house was done enough to pass its occupancy inspection and we settled in with relief, crises behind us. Or so we thought. Until one perfectly ordinary August morning three years later, when Richard saw the birds. Our days were about to get harder and more dear than we could imagine: The birds presaged a tumor growing in his right brain. A tumor that would kill him, though we didn't know that then and didn't believe it for far longer than the data warranted. The human capacity for optimistic denial is astonishing and persistent—as demonstrated by America's slow response to the coronavirus pandemic, and the mess Earth is in now.

Our impending parting was what took us to the Nature Conservancy's Carpenter Ranch in northwestern Colorado on that September day. It was the first night of our twenty-nine-years-belated honeymoon, a road trip from our Colorado home to the Pacific coast and along that wild edge from Puget Sound to Big Sur.

We hadn't had time or money for a honeymoon when we fell in love in graduate school. By the time we got as far as dreaming up a list of potential honeymoon destinations, Molly had left for college, Richard had traded academia for consulting and then sculpture, and I had written seven books. We were happy, holding hands wherever we went—secure in our belief that we had many years ahead together.

And then came the morning when my love saw those thousands of birds, tiny birds on each blade of grass, huge birds on the rims of distant mesas. Richard had always watched birds, fascinated by their flight and forms. The avian multitudes he saw that quiet morning were hallucinations—winged messengers manifested by the deadliest form of brain tumors, glioblastoma—and our reminder that our "forever" pledge was finite. Those birds sent us on a grueling journey through brain surgeries, radiation, chemotherapy, and eventually, on our honeymoon, a celebration of the love we had nurtured through it all.

No one with an ounce of sense would set off on a three-week road trip with a guy whose brain was being commandeered by a growing tumor. You'd have to be crazy with love, and also an incurable optimist who believes that time and compassion heal all wounds. That's me.

That night at Carpenter Ranch, as Richard slept beside me, I lay awake, hearing bats fluttering outside and reviewing the route ahead: the two-day drive across Wyoming, Idaho, and Oregon and into Washington, ending in Olympia with my family for the weekend. After that, following the coast south, we'd stop here and there at favorite places before spending a weekend in San Francisco with Molly. From there, we'd wind down wild Big Sur before turning inland for home. And then we'd begin another journey, our final one together: Richard's hospice care.

Driving four thousand miles in three weeks had seemed reasonable when we planned the trip in our living room. Now I wondered if I was nuts. I would be driver, guide, and nurse. The tumor impaired Richard's coordination—hence his difficulty with the stairs—and his bladder control. It created in his vision a left-side blind spot large enough to hide all of me. I felt at times like a sheepdog herding a cheerfully impaired elephant. But an elephant eager to make the trip!

What the hell were we thinking? Part of why we were both so determined to go was that the trip represented a return to some kind of normality, a way of reclaiming lives taken over by cancer treatment. Seeing it as a belated honeymoon was also lifting a metaphorical middle finger at fate, brain cancer and all. At heart, though, the trip was simply our way of celebrating the "body of love," as Richard called it, that we had nurtured.

A great horned owl hooted nearby: *Who-who-who?* I padded to the window to look out at a sky full of stars, then returned to bed and snuggled next to Richard's warm skin.

A haiku formed in my head, inspired by the owl and our trip. Poetry has run through my life since my earliest memories, whether of Mom singing nursery rhymes or my Scottish grandmother,

Chris, reciting Robert Burns in her best "bonny braw Scots." I turn to poetry the way I suppose some turn to prayer, as a way to express wonder and gratitude, explore what I do not understand, or comfort myself when the vastness of existence becomes overwhelming. I write a haiku every day to practice attention, both to individual words and to the stream of moments that make up our lives. Hence the verse taking shape as I succumbed to sleep:

*owl hoots, unanswered*
*lonely? I wonder*
*speaking only to a dazzle of stars*

# chapter two

❧

## Day Two

## Odometer Reading: 204 Miles

Our first stop the next day was our friend Terry's bookstore and coffee shop in Craig, the heart of northwest Colorado's oil patch. We lingered over my cocoa and Richard's pungent americano, talking about books and art and life. When it was time for us to hit the road for our night's stop at a favorite hot spring in Idaho, Terry traced a back-road shortcut on our map, a route that would take us by petroglyphs I had long wanted to show Richard.

As Terry escorted us to our car, Richard walked straight into a low-hanging street-tree branch with a *thunk*.

"I didn't see it," he said, as I checked his forehead: just a scrape, no lump.

"It was on your left side." I felt guilty. It was only the second day of our trip, and already I had failed to anticipate an obstacle. Some shepherd I was proving to be. "I'm sorry."

"I'm okay. My head's hard."

"That's certainly true." He grinned—as I had hoped—at my tart tone.

Terry hugged us, tears in his eyes.

Richard, who until brain surgery number four had invariably commandeered the driver's seat, climbed into the passenger side without complaint. I had mixed feelings about that change: It was a relief to be able to drive without an argument. I just hated the reason. We didn't realize then—though perhaps we should have, or at least I, who was still of intact brain, should have—that Richard's tumor growth was accelerating. In our time on the road, his brain function would deteriorate dramatically, challenging us both.

We were simply naively happy to be off on an adventure, traveling hand in hand as we had for so many miles over the years. Road trips were our best escapes. No matter where we were headed or what the reason, many of our most insightful conversations and richest shared silences had come while watching the landscapes of North America roll by the car windows, holding hands. Isn't that the American dream: car as personal magic carpet, redemption beckoning around the next bend? (Of course, car as contributor to climate change as well, which is why we now drove a compact SUV, instead of my beloved truck.)

As a child growing up in an eccentric family, I lived for hitting the road. Our family vacations were an escape from the suburbs and my schoolmates' teasing about my unfashionable clothes, our family's homemade camper van, the sack lunches my brother, Bill, and I toted to school, and Dad's habit of biking to work, lab coat flying. That camper was my winged horse, my portal to the halcyon wild.

We would pile into the van on a Friday evening. Dad drove; Mom, chief navigator, sat next to him with her magnifying glass and road maps. Bill and I lounged on opposite sides of the dinette and read, played cards, or bickered as the world rolled by the windows. Dinner would be squishy white-bread sandwiches with lunch meat and crunchy leaf lettuce from our backyard vegetable garden. After dark, Bill and I crawled into our bunks; Mom sang until the thrum of the tires lulled us to sleep. In the morning, we never knew where we would wake. It might be an expanse of wind-rippled prairie, a valley bounded by peaks spearing the sky, or a coastal cliff. Like books, those trips transported me into a world of wonder.

Richard, Molly, and I took our first family road trip the day after we married, setting out for West Virginia in a hatchback crammed with our belongings. That drive wasn't much of a vacation, but it was an adventure, a lighting-out for the unknown of Richard's first academic post in an unfamiliar landscape. After that, our family trips occurred mostly in rental trucks as we moved from place to place following his career.

Whenever we did manage a vacation, though, we found the road trip enchantment. Like the winter-break drive to Arizona to visit my parents when Mom woke us in the wee hours to watch the huge and starry blossoms of her night-blooming cereus cactus open in the moonlight. Another time, Dad showed Molly how to carefully untangle a house finch from the mist net of his banding station and then, holding the feathered form gently between her thumb and fingers, weigh and measure the small body. After he fastened a numbered aluminum tracking band around one leg, Dad let Molly release the finch. Joy filled her face as life winged from her hand.

When Richard saw the birds, he and I were on the road, bound for an artist-writer residency we had been awarded at a remote cabin in Colorado's San Juan Mountains.

As we headed to Durango to buy supplies the morning we were to begin our sojourn, he suddenly said, "What's with all the birds?"

The sky was clear, the morning air still, astringent with dust and hinting at heat to come. I scanned the high-desert landscape. The limbs of the nearby piñon pines and junipers were empty.

"What birds?" I asked, my tone carefully neutral.

"On the wires." Richard pointed at utility wires overhead. "On the branches of the willows by the pond, on the stems of the rabbitbrush." He turned in the driver's seat. "Don't you see them?"

A chill skittered down my bare arms. I looked again, searching with eyes trained by growing up in a birdwatching family. "No."

My levelheaded, logical love began describing birds on the fence posts, birds crowding the barbed wire itself; birds perched on every tree branch, on flowers along the roadside; birds on each blade of grass. Birds I could not see.

"Pull over and show me one," I said, forcing a calm I did not feel.

Although I long ago traded fieldwork for writing, I still see the world through the lens of science. It is second nature to me to observe, record, and look for patterns that explain the data. In that moment with Richard's legions of invisible birds, I was searching for a hypothesis, a comprehensible explanation for his suddenly altered reality.

He stopped the car on the dusty shoulder and put his bucket cap over the elegant skull he had begun shaving when his bald spot grew larger than his remaining hair. He walked with his usual grace, a physical man at home in his body, to a chicory plant with flowers like small blue dandelions. An exotic weed, my inner plant biologist noted. He pointed to a bird he saw.

"Touch it," I said.

Richard stretched out his hand—thumb and long fingers extended—ready to cradle its feathered body the way my father had taught Molly years before. Only Richard's fingers passed through empty air.

There was no bird.

He turned to look at me, his warm-toned skin suddenly ashen.

I got out of the car and wrapped my arms around him, his chin resting on the top of my head. Tears dripped into my hair as he described avian flocks, from fingernail-size birds perched on the gravel in the road to giant ones on distant mesas. His body shook, and I shook too, only inside, my world quaking as the man I so often leaned on now leaned on me.

Richard's affinity for birds gave my family no small amount of amusement when they realized that I, the lone nonbirdwatcher in our small flock, had fallen in love with a guy who, on our only date, quizzed me about the house finches nesting outside his office window.

I enjoy birds; they're just not my life's passion. As I have maintained since childhood, when I was periodically dragged out of bed before dawn to trek to some sewage lagoon where a rare red-legged hoo-ha had been seen, birds get up too early and, unlike plants, they don't hold still so you can easily identify them. My affinity for plants goes deep: I'm a botanist who restores habitat, a gardener rooted in tending soil and place.

"What should we do?" Richard asked.

I needed time to think. I swiped tears from my eyes, marshaled confidence I did not feel, and took a deep breath. "Let's get breakfast. Food always helps."

He pulled a handkerchief out of the back pocket of his jeans, mopped his face, and handed the cloth to me, dry end up. Then he headed for the driver's seat.

"I'll drive," I said quickly, my voice trembling with fear I would not admit.

He looked at me for a long moment and then nodded. I exhaled.

The birds followed us to town.

When the facade of the world as we thought we knew it crumbles, how we cope falls along somewhat predictable lines: curl up and pretend nothing is wrong (denial); turn and look the other way (another form of denial); continue on as if nothing happened (denial again); or perhaps take a metaphoric step or two backward and simply observe, as I did (denial as science).

Denial is a way of therapeutic stalling, allowing our subconscious to get over the shock when change wallops our lives. Stalling helps us process and figure out how to respond. But denial is dangerous when it becomes habitual, when we retreat into what a therapist friend calls "medicating and masking"—drinking to excess, dulling our pain with drugs, sex, food, religion, or whatever our preferred numbing agent is. Ignoring facts until they become a crisis of global proportions. Then we are in some deep shit.

I simply needed time to absorb the shock that Richard was suddenly seeing things—and not just any things, but birds. What could these visions mean?

After breakfast and some discussion, we aborted the residency we had been looking forward to for months and returned home, I in the driver's seat and Richard's birds traveling along. The landscape was alive with avian forms only he could see.

When we got home and settled into our sculptor-built house with its concrete floor patterned like the earth, flagstone shelves, and art by friends and family hanging on colorful walls, it no longer felt like a refuge. Richard's birds had shaken our reality.

"I can see details I never noticed before," he said. "As if the world is different."

My skin crawled. I squeezed his hand but couldn't trust my voice.

Like so many physical men, Richard rarely admitted weakness. He brushed off injuries or illnesses, whether the cuts and abrasions from sculpting granite, or colds and flu. I wonder if the only way his body could get his attention was through visions.

I called my brother for comfort and poured out the story.

Bill, a fisheries biologist and a birdwatcher of some renown, asked what kind of birds.

"Ha ha." I repeated the question to Richard.

He grinned and gestured for the phone. "They looked like red-winged blackbirds, but in different sizes."

"Too bad." My brother's voice carried. "Next time, make sure to see something interesting so I can add it to my Colorado list."

Tears rolled down my face as Richard's laugh rumbled from deep in his chest.

And now, two years, one week, and four brain surgeries later, we were on another route and I was again at the wheel. We zipped along rural two-lane roads on Terry's shortcut. Cool air poured in the open car windows, saturated with the sweet turpentine fragrance of big sagebrush, a shrub that colors and scents vast expanses of the inland West and says home to me. Buttes striped by rust, purple, olive, and ocher rock layers sprouted all around. I spotted a trio of pronghorn bucks close enough that we could hear their breathy snorts and barking warnings.

We stopped and walked uphill to the petroglyph site, a tumble of angular boulders at the base of a sheer mahogany cliff overlooking miles of open landscape. The dark rocks were scribed with pale outlines of bighorn sheep, pronghorn like the ones we had just seen, geometric masks, and the spirals of exploding nebulas. The strikingly modern images recalled the Fremont people who had carved them centuries before, a culture vanished but for the haunting rock art.

A rock wren trilled nearby, notes ringing.

"Like a hammer striking granite," Richard said.

"Like you sculpting a basin in a boulder."

"Yes, like me." Richard threw back his head and laughed, arms upraised in his habitual expression of joy. "I'm a lucky guy."

As we walked hand in hand downhill, I blessed the day. We were together, cocooned in the car, traveling through landscapes we loved. What could go wrong?

*Pronghorn barks*
*breath slapping air in a sudden "huff!"—*
*danger!*

# chapter three

## Day Two

### Odometer Reading: 311 Miles

An hour later, Richard announced, "I have to pee."

We were stopped in a queue for construction on a two-lane road in the middle of nowhere, with no building, porta potty, tree, or even sagebrush shrub to hide behind.

"It's urgent," he added, beginning to squirm.

Just then, our line of vehicles started to creep forward. "Can you wait until I find a side road?"

"I'll try."

By the time we located a turnoff, it was too late. I parked and helped him peel off his jeans and briefs, and then wet a washcloth. While he sponge-bathed, I dug out dry clothes and transferred the contents of his pockets: card case, folding knife, handkerchief, miscellaneous screws and bolts, folded dollar bills, coins, and half a dozen special pebbles. *No wonder his jeans pockets wear out so quickly,* I thought. I sighed and rolled my shoulders, releasing tension.

*Ki-YEER!* A red-tailed hawk called from overhead. Richard's face turned upward, tracking the soaring buteo, a smile bathing his features. I smiled too, watching him.

While he dressed, I took out the picnic basket and sliced bread, cheese, and an avocado for sandwiches. Soon we were on our way again, munching lunch and watching for migrating hawks and fall wildflowers. Another adaptation: Pee-soaked jeans no longer rated as a crisis.

The day after Richard's bird hallucinations, he announced that he was fine. He argued, very much the successful expert witness, when I insisted he see our family doctor. "You promised," I reminded him. I won.

Dr. Mary Reeves listened intently as Richard recounted the story, her face serious, fingers tapping the keys of her laptop. He finished by asserting again that he was "fine."

I looked at him and cleared my throat. Mary, a personal friend, scanned us over her glasses, face amused. I nudged Richard's foot. He shot me a frustrated glance.

"Susan thinks I can't recognize faces," he said. "People don't appear the same, it's true. But I can figure out who they are through contextual clues: gait, body shape, voice, dress."

"Or by asking me . . ." My tone was tart. "When we were looking in the bathroom mirror this morning, do you remember what you said when I asked if you recognized my face?"

"'You appear different than you did last week.'" Richard repeated and reached for my hand. "'But you look beautiful.'"

I blinked back tears. Mary's fingers danced over the keyboard.

"Am I crazy? Is this schizophrenia?" Richard asked.

I stared at him, shocked. For one long moment, I did not recognize the man I loved.

Mary said calmly, "If it were psychosis, you'd be arguing that the birds were real." She continued, "What you're telling me is consistent with three possibilities: damage from heat exhaustion, some unexplained neurological storm, or a mass growing in your brain."

He smiled, and he was Richard and I was me again.

Eight days later, we were on the road to Denver, a three-hour drive over the mountains, for Richard's appointment at the neurology department of the regional VA medical center. In the interim, I had watched him closely for more symptoms—and felt traitorous for that scrutiny. Over the decades, we had come to trust each other enough to discuss pretty much everything (except money, which he preferred to ignore; I handled our finances). Now, I observed Richard carefully without telling him, in effect collecting data without his knowledge, a violation of our implicit agreement that any problem was solvable if shared.

I was simply turning to the same careful observation I used for my own health. When I was diagnosed with lupus at age twenty-three and told I likely had only a few years to live, I employed my science training: I read the research on the incurable condition, took notes on the occurrence and frequency of my symptoms, looked for patterns in the data, and adapted my life to stay as healthy as possible. Observation was key, and is still one of my best tools. I assumed Richard wouldn't mind my using those methods on him. But I didn't ask.

Assumptions like that are the shorthand of life, unspoken premises we rely on to simplify our days. They shape our roles and interactions, our biases and beliefs, for good or ill. One of Richard's and my primary assumptions—one that shaped our collective decisions, from who would be the main breadwinner to where we would live—was that he was healthy and I was not. Brain cancer proved us wrong. Unexamined, assumptions become straitjackets we chafe against at best, and at worst, positively dangerous, like the assumptions that once we "beat" the novel coronavirus, life will return to normal, or that humans have some divine mandate to exploit this planet for our benefit.

It was dusk on the belated honeymoon trip, and we were still almost an hour from our night's destination when we stopped so Richard could pee for what seemed to me like the millionth time that day. While he emptied his bladder, I unwrapped his favorite road-trip dinner: an egg-and-potato burrito with green chile sauce. He ate happily while I drove on, exhausted from the effort to be chauffeur, navigator, and herder of a man whose left brain might still be brilliant but whose right had serious issues, including perceiving signals from his bladder.

Chile sauce suddenly exploded all over the steering wheel, the dashboard, and Richard.

"Damn it!" I shouted. "I'm doing everything! Can't you at least eat without making a bloody mess?"

I pulled over, took a breath, and rubbed my gritty eyes. I reminded myself that the tumor was the problem, not Richard.

He pulled himself out of the car, face a study in misery, chile sauce dripping down his shirt. I touched his shoulder. "I'm sorry, sweetie. Forgive me." I fetched a washcloth and cleaned Richard and then the car.

As I drove on, we agreed on road trip rule number one: no messy food in a moving car. It was pragmatic, an acknowledgment of the seismic shift in our roles initiated by the bird hallucinations and what we had learned at his first neurology appointment, two years before.

Richard held the glass door of the medical center open for me. We wound our way through the halls hand in hand and climbed six flights of stairs. The Neurology waiting room was crowded, but we nabbed two seats together. I opened my laptop, doing my best to ignore the blaring television, a skill I never entirely perfected. Richard read an art book.

Finally, a voice called, "Richard Cabe?" A serious-faced, dark-haired young woman wearing a white physician's coat shook our hands. She introduced herself as Sarah Kuykendall, a neurology resident.

"What brings you in today?" she asked when we were settled in the small exam room.

Richard told the story of the bird hallucinations; I chimed in with details he left out.

Dr. Kuykendall listened, took notes, and administered a neurological exam, the first of so many that eventually Richard could run through the test without prompting. He passed easily.

She asked if he used street drugs or alcohol. He smiled. "No drugs. I've never wanted to make myself stupid. I do drink one Belgian-style ale every day, without fail."

Dr. Kuykendall chuckled, tapped her teeth with a pen, and then asked us to wait while she talked to her attending physician.

When she left, Richard patted his lap. We snuggled, arms around each other, talking quietly, and then fell silent. I looked out the window at a rooftop garden and tried to empty my mind of worries. I wished I had spent more time learning human biology. I'm a field ecologist fascinated by the relationships between species that weave whole landscapes. Lab work is not my thing. I've never peered into the microworld of cells, or studied brain synapses and neurons.

Dr. Kuykendall returned with Dr. Filley, a slender man wearing a jacket and tie. He grinned as I uncurled myself from Richard's lap. He shook our hands, then scanned the notes. "I know you've been all through this with Dr. Kuykendall, but I'd like to hear the story in your own words. Both your words." His smile included me. (Richard's team always included me; the VA explicitly recognizes how important families and caregivers are in supporting the patient's treatment.)

Richard launched into the tale again. I amended. Dr. Filley listened, stroking his clean-shaven chin. "Your symptoms don't qualify you for an emergency MRI," he said when Richard finished, "but we need to know what's going on." He grinned. "The head of radiology owes me a favor. I'm going to give him a call."

The two docs left. I moved back to the comfort of Richard's lap. After a while, Dr. Kuykendall returned and let us know the MRI department could fit us in.

"And afterward?" I asked. "Can we drive home?"

"By all means. We'll call in a day or two with the results."


By midafternoon, we were headed across the city, toward the mountains and home, Richard at the wheel, when his cell phone buzzed. He handed it to me.

"Susan? This is Sarah Kuykendall in Neurology at the VA. Is Richard driving?"

Goose bumps skittered down my arms, "Yes."

"Tell him to pull over."

*Shit.* I covered the phone. "It's Dr. Kuykendall. Find a place to park, okay?"

Richard turned onto a side street and stopped in the shade of an elm tree. I aimed the phone so he could hear it.

"I'm sorry, but we need to admit Richard to the hospital. His MRI shows severe inflammation and a lesion in the right temporal lobe." Dr. Kuykendall explained that was the area responsible for processing visual stimuli, hence his hallucinations. She asked if we had questions.

I couldn't think. My was mind stuck on Richard's going to the hospital. That was so wrong. Sitting next to me in the car, with the sleeves of his pressed blue oxford shirt rolled back to reveal tanned and muscled forearms, he looked his robust self. Yet the MRIs showed devastating inflammation and a lesion—whatever that meant—in his right brain.

After the call, we discussed the facts. But I couldn't articulate my emotions: stunned terror at the idea of our being parted, he in a hospital bed, I in a motel. I felt guilty, as if by covertly observing Richard I had drawn a line that split "us," two people so close that we often finished each other's sentences and friends referred to us as the collective "Richard 'n' Susan," instead of by our individual names. A line that implied we *could* be parted.

I felt Richard's warm hand in mine. I heard a sprinkler hissing from a nearby lawn, the swish of car tires passing, the tuneless chatter of house sparrows. I looked sideways at his handsome face, hazel eyes clear, watching a robin probe for a worm in a nearby lawn.

*It's like a bad dream. Only I am awake and terrified. I have a sense of something dreadfully wrong, but I can't find words to describe it.*

"We never sleep apart," I finally said. "How will we manage?"

"We'll be okay, my love." He pulled me close and kissed me. "We'll be okay."

Later, he called Molly while I called my parents. I heard Molly's worried voice: "Should I come?"

"No, sweetie." Richard's tone was soothing. "I'm fine."


At the hot springs that second night of our honeymoon trip, we drifted hand in hand in steaming water as pinprick stars appeared in the sky overhead. Floating on my back, I pointed when the full moon rose, silver-bright. "Look!"

Richard squinted, cajoling his impaired vision to resolve detail from the darkness, and slowly smiled. "There's our moon." He pulled me in for a kiss, his lips warm and sweet.

*the moon!*
*full round, swimming among stars*
*we drift below, hand in hand*

Later, as I snuggled next to my snoring love, I was swamped with guilt for having lost my temper at him over the chile explosion. I took a long breath and reminded myself that I didn't have to be perfect; I simply had to be the best me I could in any given moment.

Being perfect is not the human condition. Nor should it be—
if we were perfect, we couldn't stumble and fail and thus learn and
grow. The failures may be hard to forgive ourselves for, but they
teach us the most. And that learning helps us grow into our best
selves. If anything demands those best selves, it's seeing death
ahead—or the world in crisis, doom inexorably approaching like
the headlight of an oncoming train. That pitiless light either para-
lyzes us or opens new insights. Or both, at different times. How
we respond is our own choice.

Richard and I chose to respond with love. Love for each other
and Molly, love for the village of friends and family who sheltered
us, love for the earth and its whole community of lives, the miracle
that quickens this blue planet. Recognizing that our love wasn't
perfect. That we would also respond with anger, guilt, and fear.
Knowing that love couldn't heal all wounds, but it could carry us
through.

# chapter four

## Day Three

### Odometer Reading: 503 Miles

"Are we going all the way to Pendleton?" Richard asked, as he settled into the car the next morning.

"That's the plan," I said. "It's a long drive. But then tomorrow we'll have time to dawdle on the scenic route in the gorge and still make it to Olympia in time for dinner."

"Okay," he said, reclining his seat. "Don't get a speeding ticket."

I laughed. "I don't have the lead foot—that's you." Richard had once gotten nabbed going fifteen miles over the speed limit after spotting one of his favorite birds—*Xanthocephalus xanthocephalus*, the yellow-headed blackbird.

"I'll keep an eye out for the highway patrol," he offered.

He was asleep by the time I turned onto the interstate half an hour later. I set the cruise control, looked over at Richard's peaceful face, and remembered that first hospital stay.

It was late afternoon by the time our patient liaison, a friendly third-year medical student, called me with the news that Richard was settled in Ward 5 South. I raced up four flights of stairs, eager to see my guy. When I found his four-person room and parted the curtains around his bed, he was fast asleep. By the time his dinner tray arrived, Richard was sitting up and filling me in on his day. He was feeling good, that was clear, but the cause of his brain swelling was still a mystery.

I eyed the meal on the tray: chicken-fried chicken smothered with gravy; instant mashed potatoes and canned peas; a plastic container of waxy fruit cocktail; and another container, of chocolate pudding, whose ingredients, I would bet, contained no actual nutritional value at all. "I could bring you real food from the deli when I walk out for dinner."

Richard thought for a moment. "No. I'm going to submit wholeheartedly to the treatment my doctors recommend, and that includes eating hospital meals." Then he, who took pride in baking crusty whole wheat boule, poked the slice of squishy white bread and added, "Except, perhaps, for the bread."

I opened my mouth to protest. Over the decades, I've learned the hard way that no matter how good it tastes, high-fat and highly processed food like what was on Richard's dinner tray is not healthy—for me or for the planet. But then I shut my mouth. Experience has also taught me that health is an individual thing we sort out for ourselves. My role was to support Richard's decisions unless I thought he was endangering himself.

When I met Richard and Molly, I was still struggling to understand how to manage my lupus. I had just begun to grasp that when I felt good about myself, my health improved. That shouldn't be a surprise, but after Western culture divorced mind from body during the postmedieval Age of Reason, we stopped believing in the power of emotions to affect our health. When seventeenth-century French philosopher René Descartes asserted, "*Cogito, ergo sum*" ("I am thinking, therefore I exist"), his words implied that who we are is all in our minds. He was wrong.

The connection between mind and body is so intimate and complicated that researchers are still discovering new dimensions to explore. One recent revelation is the impact of our gut micro-biome—the billions of microscopic creatures who live in our intestines—on our state of mind. We now know that those minute flora and fauna have a profound impact on our emotions and overall mental health by producing compounds that act on our brains. Moreover, the relationship works both ways: Our brains affect gastrointestinal and immune functions that can shape which microbe species survive in the gurgling stew in our guts, and thus which brain-influencing chemicals they release. Feeling good about ourselves, or cultivating a positive attitude, it seems, can truly make us healthier via that microbial connection. That connection also means we are not the rugged individuals we like to imagine; each of us is shaped by our teeming internal communities. Think about that: If I am not "me" alone—if I, in science writer Ed Yong's words "contain multitudes"—who am I? It's impossible to ignore the implication: We are not "above" or alienated from nature; our microbial ecosystems make us very much part of this planet's living web.

At seven thirty the next morning, after Richard was moved to a single room, I sat in the visitor's chair, feet on the bed rails, drinking my hot chocolate and typing on my laptop. Richard sat cross-legged on the bed, sipping the aromatic dark-roast coffee I had brought him and writing in a breast pocket–size notebook that served both as journal and as sculpture sketchbook.

Dr. Allen ("Call me Brooke"), the head neurology resident, knocked on the open door.

"Do you want to see the MRI images?" She smiled as she pushed curling brown hair away from her face.

Did we ever! We followed her down the hall to a computer at the nurses' station.

I had never seen an MRI before, so it took me a few beats to make sense of the reversed cross-sections. The jutting outline at the top was Richard's nose, the rounded curve at the bottom was the back of his skull; his right brain was on the left side of the screen.

The difference between the two halves was dramatic and chilling: The left displayed a gorgeous, symmetrical fractal architecture: in-branching folds between the lobes, plus the open ovals of the vesicles where fluid circulated. The right was a featureless blob, swollen as a sausage in its casing. As I looked at it, my stomach roiled and I swayed, suddenly dizzy. I reached for Richard's hand.

Brooke was pointing to a white area in Richard's right temporal lobe. "Something damaged your brain there. We don't know what. When we first looked at this MRI, we couldn't conceive how you were functioning. Most people with this kind of brain swelling present in a coma, hooked up to a ventilator. Yet there you were, walking, talking, apparently fully functional except for the visual hallucinations. Your left brain took over, and brilliantly. You're very lucky."

As Richard and I walked hand in hand back to his room, those images played over in my mind: the left hemisphere with its graceful, curvilinear geometry, the right so swollen it was a miracle Richard was upright, able to hold my hand and walk briskly in hospital bed socks.

I couldn't reconcile the images with the guy who passed his hospital time solving sudoku puzzles, reading dense books about art theory, precisely forming paper into models of abstract sculptures, and watching birds out the window. Sitting cross-legged on the bed, with his metal-framed reading glasses perched on his nose, high cheekbones, shaved head, and closely trimmed silver beard, Richard looked, as one staffer put it, "like Gandhi in hospital pajamas." Except Gandhi didn't have a lesion in his right brain.

*Gandhi*, in which Ben Kingsley stars as Mohandas Gandhi, was our first film date. After we dropped Molly at preschool one afternoon, Richard said, "Want to play hooky and see a movie?"

I had writing deadlines and women's center work; he had comprehensive exams to prepare for and student assignments to grade. "Absolutely!" I said.

We bought a pizza, and Richard nonchalantly smuggled the box into the theater under his sheepskin jacket, without letting go of my hand. By the end of the movie, I was in tears, swept up in the emotions and injustice; Richard, ever the intellectual, was fired up by Gandhi's ideas.

Over the next few days at the hospital, groups of students, residents, and medical staff passed through Richard's room while the docs discussed his still-mysterious case. (The Denver VA hospital serves as a teaching facility for the University of Colorado School of Medicine.) Whenever anyone asked about Richard's work, I opened my laptop to display photos of his sculptures. My favorite was a one-ton granite boulder he carved into a stunning fire pit. After studying the massive rock, Richard "saw" a basin nestled between two thick white quartz veins on one side. He planed that side of the boulder flat for a top, carved a bowl-shaped indentation in the center, and polished the top and the basin itself to reveal the boulder's crystalline interior. Then he hand-hammered a sheet of raw steel into a bowl and suspended it inside the polished basin to contain the flames. The rest of the boulder's exterior, he left rough, shaped by glaciers, water, and time, as if the earth itself were spouting fire.

Richard was embarrassed. "You don't need to brag about me."

I did—I wanted his team to know the person inside the hospital gown and the data. "Showing your sculpture forges a human connection," I said. "It might inspire their work."

He thought for a moment. "I'll try to live up to that."

"Just be you—that's enough."


Anything that disturbs the neural fabric of our brains alters our self-defined "us." Richard prided himself on his intellect, which survived the tumor in his right brain without diminution; it's a left-brain function. Even when his right brain could no longer make sense of a cell phone or notice an emotion, he could talk intelligently about anything, from the Buddhist concept of lovingkindness to the economic disincentive of the British land tax in Gandhi's time.

Why Richard's transitory visual hallucinations took the form of birds is not clear. Perhaps his brain's interpretation of the visual input filtered through his injured temporal lobe was biased by his interest in all things avian. When the birds disappeared after twenty-four hours, Richard assumed the crisis had passed. If I hadn't insisted he see our doctor, he wouldn't have ended up in the hospital, and, Dr. Filley said later, the brain swelling would have killed him. I am grateful for the birds; their warning gave us two more years. Difficult years, yes, but precious nonetheless.

By the time we headed off on the Big Trip, the cumulative impact of four brain surgeries, radiation, two courses of chemotherapy, and the growing tumor had altered Richard's brain function in ways I often couldn't predict. Like when he got out of the car at Farewell Bend State Recreation Area on the Snake River in eastern Oregon on day three. This place, where the river, its powerful flow deceptively placid, heads into the wild Snake River Canyon, was a favorite stop. On that hot afternoon when the car thermometer read ninety-five degrees Fahrenheit, I parked in the shade, unfolded my tired body, and stretched my back—and then watched with horror as Richard began to unzip his fly in full view of a family at a nearby picnic table. I hustled him behind a tree.

"Damn it! You can't whip out your penis in plain sight!" I hissed. "No peeing in public."

He cocked his head and asked, "Is that a rule?"

I tamped down my redhead's temper with some difficulty. "Yes. Rule number two."

He considered as his stream dwindled to a trickle, and then nodded. "That's reasonable."

I sighed. It was like dealing with a six-year-old in a sixty-one-year-old's body. *He's still with you*, I reminded myself. *Be grateful.*

Two hours later, we wound into Oregon's Blue Mountains, the last range before Pendleton. A smoky haze from distant fires colored the evening sun orange.

"Let's eat dinner with the larch trees," Richard said.

"Okay."

On our many drives to Portland, where Molly had gone to college and worked her first professional job, or Olympia, where Bill and Lucy and family lived, we always watched for the larch trees in the Blue Mountains. These unusual conifers of high-mountain and far northern forests are conspicuous when their needles turn brilliant yellow in fall and sprout tender green in spring. We had discovered a shared love of larches that long-ago winter in Laramie.

"I have something to show you," Richard announced when he arrived at the women's center to pick me up one bitterly cold February night.

I pulled on my down jacket, cap, and mittens, wound a scarf around my neck, and followed his tall form down the stairs and out into the darkness. We walked mitten in mitten past the campus library, our footsteps crunching on new snow, breath issuing silver clouds of frost.

A few blocks later, Richard stopped and pointed. "Do you recognize that tree?"

I swiped eyes watering from the cold and squinted at long, bare branches knobby with fat, pearl-like buds. "It's a larch! I didn't know they could grow here."

"It's the only one I've found in town."

I began to shiver. Richard pulled me close; we headed toward my house and warmth.

"I love you," he said later, as he stroked my breasts. "I love making love with the woman who would walk across town with me on a subzero night to admire a larch tree."

Near the summit of the Blue Mountains, I took an exit onto a quiet two-lane road that wound through the forest. I was looking for a picnic spot with larches, when Richard woke and announced, "I have to pee."

I immediately turned down a deserted logging road. Richard got out, ducked behind a tree, and said, "Hello, larch!" as he watered its trunk. I chuckled, bone-weary, and pulled out the cooler. As we picnicked side by side, a mountain chickadee sang a hoarse *Phoe-bee! Phoe-bee!*, half a dozen elk ambled past, and the almost-full moon rose.

"Chickadee, elk, moonrise, and larch trees," said Richard. "I'm a lucky guy."

Holding gratitude for the gift of what we're losing—whether a beloved person or a whole planet—in the same heart space with grief and anger is a moving equilibrium like juggling, a skill I've never mastered. Love jostles pain, opposites nestled like yin and yang, the duality at the core of existence, their boundaries shifting yet always inseparable.

> *Blue Mountain sunset*
> *bright ball vanishes in orange haze—*
> *distant fires*

# chapter five

*Day Four*

## Odometer Reading: 1,146 Miles

The next day, we reached cool, smoke-free air in the Columbia River Gorge and stopped at Hood River for lunch at Richard's favorite microbrewery. Our table overlooked the wind-ruffled surface of the wide river, cordoned by massive cliffs of dark-columned basalt stairstepping toward blue sky. Sailboarders scudded the waves; anglers fished for salmon; gulls kited the wind.

"The first time we drove this way, we were moving from Olympia to Boulder." Richard slowly licked brown-ale foam from his mustache.

I remembered that trip: Molly was nine years old; we had quit our jobs and sold our house to return to the Rockies so Richard could finish his PhD.

He forked up a bite of fresh-caught salmon. "How many times do you suppose we've driven through the gorge together?"

I counted on my fingers: that one-way trip in a U-Haul truck, towing our old Volvo; visits to Bill, Lucy, and the girls; a trip for Molly's cousin Jennifer's wedding; then taking Molly to college at

Reed and returning twice a year until she graduated. "Nearly a dozen."

He nodded. "This is likely my last trip. Thank you for bringing me."

Tears blurred my vision. I reached for his hand. "I love you."

"Love" was not just a word we traded. It was a way of living that Richard and I deliberately cultivated—our expression of both our bond and our species' terraphilia. At bedtime, we each spoke intentions aloud as part of our practice of mindfulness, a word that has become almost trite but that has real meaning. Mindfulness is simply an effort to be aware of our moment-by-moment experience and choices—of thoughts, feelings, and what goes on around us—without judgment, but with the intention of living "awake," not on autopilot. The words we spoke to each other each night were a promise to be our best selves.

Mine began with "To live with my heart outstretched as if it were my hand," a line I had adapted from a Mary Chapin Carpenter song I first heard one fall when we were driving the aspen-dappled mountains above Taos, New Mexico, on an art studio tour, Richard at the wheel, as always. As I listened to Chapin Carpenter's "Goodnight America," my ears perked up at a line about dreaming with her heart outstretched as if it were her hand.

"That's my writing mission!" I cued the song again.

Richard listened: "Not just writing. You're *living* with your heart outstretched as if it were your hand."

Richard's intention was simple: "To be a source of support and joy," he said every night, "and to live with lovingkindness."

He didn't always succeed. Nor did I. Our flaws regularly tried our intentions, even before the brain issues. Caregiving certainly tried me—patience is not my virtue, no matter the love involved.

The warrior in me rose to the challenge; the woman feared losing herself in the doing.

After four days in the hospital, Richard's brain had recovered, but the cause of his brainstorm remained a mystery. He was on track to be sent home when a visiting expert in brain viruses raised the possibility of a viral infection. Viruses are very bad news in brains —difficult to detect, swiftly fatal. The expert recommended treatment with an intravenous antiviral drug—which meant ten more days in the hospital.

"Could the infusions be delivered at home?" I asked Richard's team Thursday evening.

"That could mean you'd have to deliver them." Brooke Allen looked at me.

"I can do that." My voice sounded more confident than I felt. Richard nodded.

After some discussion, the team agreed; still, it would be Monday before Richard was released. The wheels of hospital bureaucracy grind slowly.

On rounds Friday morning, Dr. Tyler, the virus expert, mentioned that his recommendation was based on a set of prior assumptions. Richard responded that Tyler was using Bayesian decision theory, a probability theory named for eighteenth-century mathematician Thomas Bayes. Dr. Tyler looked delighted and launched into a math-geek discussion of Bayesian priors with Richard. Dr. Kuykendall rolled her eyes at me. I grinned back.

"I like proving that parts of my brain still work," Richard said later, his smile wide.

Molly flew in for the weekend, bringing sunshine with her. As I listened to Richard tell her animatedly about the twin basins he was sculpting into sinks for our master bathroom from two halves of a blue granite boulder—"One for Suz, the other for me"—my eyes filled with tears. I walked to the window at the end of the hall. Resting my forehead on the cool glass, I saw the bench across the street where Molly and Richard had sat side by side earlier, he AWOL in his blue hospital pajamas, reading glasses on, she catching up on work, laptop in her lap. Their heads were together, their smiling faces incandescent.

Walking back, Richard bent down, picked up three rocks from the ground, and began to juggle. Molly laughed. He dropped the rocks and raised his arms over his head in joy—so alive.

Richard and I had grown into, as one friend put it, "each other's other half," mirrored like those basins he was carving. He was very much the traditional guy: He analyzed, engineered, designed, and built; his work charted the path for our lives; he took the wheel on road trips. I was the nurturer, tending our household, our families, and the land. I handled the details of life "on the material plane," as he put it, like tracking expenses and paying bills. Our roles weren't always comfortable, but they were familiar. And now? What changes lay ahead?

One change was certain, and enormously difficult: my transition from being Richard's lover, partner, and best friend to being his caregiver—starting with the infusions.

After we arrived home Monday night, Marty, a tall and rangy home health care nurse, taught me how to administer Richard's infusions. First, Marty explained the supplies: Alcohol swabs to sterilize the port on Richard's PICC line, an IV line ending in an artery near his heart. Syringes filled with clear saline solution to flush the port; the yellow ones contained heparin, a blood thinner to keep clogs from forming. Canisters that looked like plastic infant-formula bottles, which were pressurized doses of acyclovir, the antiviral.

Then Marty walked me through the process: "Sterilize, flush, attach." He showed me how to sterilize the port, squirt air bubbles out of a full saline syringe, screw it into the port protruding from Richard's left forearm, push down the plunger, unscrew the empty syringe, and attach the pressurized canister to dispense the acyclovir. The infusion finished, Marty demonstrated how to flush the line with saline, inject the heparin, clean the port again, and replace the cap.

"Any questions?" he asked.

It was nine o'clock, and I was too exhausted to think. I looked at Richard. He shook his head.

"If you get stuck," Marty said, as he stowed his gear, "call the home health care number. We can be here in a few minutes."

The next morning's infusion went off without a hitch. After lunch, we hit the first snag when Richard noticed an air bubble in the line just below his port.

"We can't do the infusion," he said, voice tight. "Air bubbles are dangerous."

"I think I can suction the bubble out with a syringe."

He disagreed. The more I tried reason, the more my usually even-tempered, logical spouse dug in. "You don't know," he said, his voice knife-sharp. "You're not a nurse."

Ouch. "If you can't trust me, call the home health care agency." My inner redhead's temper flaring, I stomped outside to calm down.

When I came back, Richard was sulking. He hadn't called the nurse.

"Richard was such a sweet boy," Miss Alice, his mother, once said in a reminiscent mood. "When he wasn't stubborn," his sister, Letitia, added later. It was true: Richard was sweet, but when he dug in his heels, nothing could move him.

*If you can't move the mountain, go around it.* I picked up the phone.

Ten minutes later, the nurse on call showed me how to suck the air bubble out of the line using the saline syringe, and then watched as I started his infusion.

"You're doing a good job," she said warmly. "You're a natural."

I resisted—barely—shooting a smug *I told you so* look at Richard.

Over the next seven days and eighteen infusions, I got more or less accustomed to shooting drugs into a port that ended directly above my love's heart, where one small error could have drastic consequences. But I never became comfortable with the role or the responsibility. The balance of our relationship had tilted from "half of each other" toward caregiver and cared-for.

Caregiving is an overwhelmingly female task. Nearly a third of adults in the United States provide care for a family member; some two-thirds of those caregivers are female. We have the breasts, those organs of nurture, so apparently the role comes naturally. Not! Women are the majority of caregivers because our careers and salaries are generally the expendable ones. And, like Greta Thunberg reluctantly rising to her role as town crier for

Earth in this time of climate catastrophe, women take on caregiving simply because it must be done.

We may not have a choice about becoming caregivers—whether for this planet or for the humans we love—but we do have a choice about our attitude. My intention was always to remember to apply the "care" in caregiving, though I didn't always succeed. As I wrote in my blog, "Each time I fail, I just need to notice and take up my practice again. It's that simple, and that difficult."

Nearly two years later, we rolled onto the interstate after lunch at the microbrewery in Hood River. Richard slid a Dar Williams CD into the player and fumbled with the buttons. I asked which song he was looking for.

"The One Who Knows." He sang a few lines, but his once-sure tenor voice wobbled.

I took my eyes off the road and selected the song. Williams's soaring voice filled the car. At the end, Richard paraphrased the lyrics: "You're taking me to the mountains and to the sea. It's you who taught me how far love goes."

Which brought up rule number three: Don't make Susan cry while she's driving. That made us both laugh. Up and down went grief's seesaw of emotions.

Richard leaned his head back and closed his eyes. "Let's stop at Multnomah Falls," he said. "I want to take a picture of you."

At the falls, I sat on a low rock wall in front of the narrow ribbon of falling water. A nuthatch yammered nearby. Richard squinted one eye as he composed the photo.

"The waterfall isn't pouring into my head, is it?" I asked, half joking.

Richard grinned. Indeed, in the picture, the white waterfall pours directly into the top of my head, over my tired eyes. Rule number four: Have a sense of humor. You'll need it.

"Did you know you were going to add 'infusion tech' to your résumé?" Richard joked, as I set up the supplies for his second-to-last day of infusions. It was my fifty-third birthday. He hadn't mentioned the day, and I was hurt but too stubborn to bring it up. I swallowed a bubble of resentment as I focused on squirting an air bubble out of the saline syringe, then flushed his line and attached the canister. "Honestly, while I love you, infusion tech is not my dream job."

He laughed. I didn't.

I turned away. He pulled me back into a hug with his free arm. "Happy birthday! I'm a fortunate guy to have you in my life."

I closed my eyes before the tears fell.

"Let's test your new inflatable kayak this afternoon," he said, "That's celebratory."

I took a deep breath. I was behind on writing deadlines and everything else. But playing hooky to try out the double kayak he had bought me was tempting. "After I finish writing my newspaper column."

Late that afternoon, we drove to a small lake at the edge of town. It was a balmy Indian-summer day, sunny and warm, with a light breeze. Richard unpacked and inflated the kayak, a complicated process that involved half filling one chamber and then the others in a specific order.

And then, putting on his life vest, he paused, looking down, one hand holding each side, his expression puzzled, as if he had no clue how to work the zipper. Watching him, I shivered, suddenly fearful. How could a simple zipper confuse the brain that could build a house, outwit an attorney in cross-examination, solve a complex math equation, or sculpt a boulder?

The moment passed. Richard zipped up the vest. We slid into the kayak; he took the stern, I the bow. A woodpecker drummed on a nearby cottonwood limb as we pushed off. After a few strokes, our paddling rhythm synchronized and we began to play. We paddled for an hour, until a cloud building over the peaks began to shoot out lightning bolts, sending us smartly back to shore, still grinning.

Time in nature heals. That shouldn't surprise us, since the living community that inspires our terraphilia is also our species' natal home. Research confirms the beneficial effects of "vitamin N": lower blood pressure and heart rates, reduced production of the stress hormone cortisol, improved mood (nature even alleviates depression), faster and more complete healing, and increased ability to focus and learn. No wonder I run off to wild country in difficult times. Time out from the busyness of the human world reweaves us, body, mind, and spirit.

The evening of our fourth day on the Big Trip, we lounged in the shade of my sister-in-law, Lucy's, kiwi arbor while she, Bill, and their youngest, Alice, cracked open the shells of fresh Dungeness crab Bill had brought home. Richard ate the succulent meat slowly, with concentration. Then, setting down a half-picked crab leg, he took a sip of beer and leaned back, eyes closed.

I watched, concerned. "Do you want me to pick out the meat?"

"No." His voice was content. "I'm just taking in this moment, full of fresh crab and love."

Bill put an arm around my shoulder. Lucy wiped her eyes. Alice looked sad. Richard opened his eyes, smiled, and picked up the crab leg again.

Savor the moment. That was rule number five, and perhaps the most important.

*hot evening*
*kiwi vine throws cool shade*
*we savor each other*

## chapter six

❧

*Day Six*

### Odometer Reading: 1,458 Miles

The next afternoon, the entire Washington Tweit clan gathered at Bill and Lucy's. The air rang with children's shouts as the four youngest—three boys and one girl, their self-appointed leader—chased each other through the house and yard.

Richard sat in the shade, beaming, a Belgian ale in his hand. As I whizzed past to set a platter of salmon burgers on the kids' table, he pulled me close. "Sit with me for a minute."

I resisted, caught up in doing. And then I remembered the point of this trip: to celebrate being together. Because we could no longer pretend—as humans are wont to do—that our "together" would last forever. I sat, platter and all.

Richard took my hand. "Thank you for sharing your family with me and Molly."

I wiped my eyes. "They loved you from the first." I kissed him. "Who wouldn't?"

My eldest niece, Heather, heard the exchange and gulped a sob through her smile.

It took me decades to understand how the differences in our families had shaped us. Richard and I share white, middle-class backgrounds, but that's about it. Take family size: My clan is tiny, a tribe of four—Mom, Dad, Bill, and me—and thus tightly bonded. (My parents were both only children; I have no aunts, uncles, or cousins.) Richard's family, by contrast, is sprawling and not always close: between them, his parents had eight siblings. Whenever Miss Alice, Richard's mother, pulled out family photos, I longed for a map to trace who belonged to whom. Miss Alice got lost too, and sometimes even confused her four kids.

And then there's culture. Arkansas, I learned on my first visit to Richard's folks, views itself as part of the South. It was clear immediately that my people are from what my in-laws consider the wrong side of the Mason-Dixon line: New Jersey (Dad) and California (Mom). Our views on everything from race and religion to environment and politics were . . . different. I learned to listen for commonalities, a practice we desperately need in these polarized times.

The thing that troubled me most was what wasn't said. I never heard any of Richard's family members use the word "love"—until our last visit to Arkansas, when Richard was dying. As we parted, his mother said, "I love you, son." Perhaps because my clan is small, we love generously and out loud. We stay in touch, hug fiercely, and say "I love you" always. It's who we are.

That Sunday in Olympia, the clan was missing only Molly, whom we would visit in San Francisco, and Dad, back at home in Colorado. I worried about how he was doing on his own.

A decade before, Dad and Mom had been happily settled in

Tucson. The Kids, as we called them, for their energy and enthusi-
asm, were active hikers, birdwatchers, and native-plant gardeners.
They volunteered as naturalists in national parks and monuments
throughout the West. Then, just before Dad's seventieth birthday,
the man who could spot a hawk when it was just a dot in the sky
lost almost two-thirds of his field of view to glaucoma. Along with
that vision loss went Dad's driver's license and their mobility.
(Mom, born completely color-blind and quite nearsighted, had
never learned to drive.)

For two years, the Kids got around via Tucson's sketchy bus
system, and then decided to move to a place with better mass
transit, and nearer to one of their kids. We toured them around
Denver on a July weekend that seemed horrendously hot to we
who are mountain dwellers but that felt pleasant to my desert-rat
parents. They found an apartment they liked and, six weeks later,
Bill drove them north and we unpacked and settled them in. Mom
and Dad explored their new neighborhood on foot, and took the
bus and light rail on farther expeditions. They were delighted to
find they could "bus" to mountain trailheads and go hiking—my
silver-haired, blue-eyed mom, her body shrunken and twisted by
rheumatoid arthritis, leading my tall, smiling, and now legally
blind dad into more adventures.

"The Kids" also referred to my parents' toddler-style insis-
tence that they could do everything themselves, thank you very
much. Only they really no longer could. Which left me, their de-
fault caregiver, to divine and provide the assistance they were sure
they didn't need. I reminded myself frequently that at least I
wasn't beginning the journey of aging-parent care while I still had
kids at home to tend to, as is the case for many of my friends in
our so-called sandwich generation. As many as one in eight Amer-

icans between the ages of forty and sixty care for aging parents while raising children or grandchildren. Managing that dual caregiver role seemed impossible to me, until Richard's birds carried us into the world of brain cancer and there I was, sandwiched between my husband and my parents. I felt trapped. Feeling trapped with no way out may explain why we cling to denial, whether about the seriousness of health issues, our national situation, or global crises.

"This is what worries us." Brooke Allen pointed at a chalk-white outline starkly visible in the latest MRI images.

We were back at the VA medical center for Richard's postinfusion checkup. Brooke had greeted us with hugs and delight at how healthy Richard looked. She asked how he felt. "Good," he said.

I was relieved to see that the two halves of Richard's brain were again symmetrical, showing the beautiful, dichotomous branching pattern so like river systems or plant veins. The curvilinear lines reminded me of his abstract sculpture, evoking the earth he loved.

Then Brooke pointed to that outline, a circle that stood out flat white against the sparkly gray of healthy tissue in his right temporal lobe, where the swelling had caused the bird hallucinations. She flipped through the images. The ghostly outline grew larger and then smaller, like a globe nesting in his brain.

"It suggests a tumor."

I reached for Richard's hand.

"It could just be a scar from the infection. I've sent the images to Dr. Tyler, to Dr. Brega in Neurosurgery, and to a neuro-oncologist . . ."

Neuro-oncologist: neuro—"of the brain"—oncologist; a cancer doctor. Brain cancer.

I forced myself to inhale, exhale, and focus, pushing away the clutch of fear. I needed to be present and remember details. Details are crucial in medical treatment, which is one reason I accompanied Richard to every appointment. (The other was, of course, for support.)

Everyone needs an advocate—someone who has our back, who listens and takes notes, who asks questions we don't think of. Who isn't blinded by emotion. (I struggle with that part.) Advocates are crucial to successful medical treatment, and also to healing and restoring our communities and this planet. We can all be advocates in our own ways, if we work together.

"We're working with Neurosurgery to schedule a biopsy as soon as possible." In the best case, Brooke said, the circular shape was scar tissue; next best, it was a tumor but benign; next no so best, it was a slow-growing brain cancer that could be treated without surgery. "In the worst case . . ." She paused. "You're healthy. We're all hoping for the best."

Richard's gaze was fixed on the MRI image with that telling circle. I looked around the windowless space, desperate for some reassuring aliveness: a glimpse of autumn-blue sky, the sound of a house finch's warbling. I saw dingy walls; I heard the tuneless beep of a telephone.

"I'll let you know as soon as I hear anything," Brooke said.

That night, I lay awake beside my sleeping love, recalling a conversation a few weeks after we met that illuminated my attraction to Richard. It wasn't his sculpted good looks, or even his mind, though I admired his intellect. My heart had surrendered to the man who loved the earth the way I did. (Much later, I realized that while my terraphilia was rooted in a specific geography, his was abstract, intellectual.) We sat in my fourth-floor office at the University of Wyoming, watching the distant peaks of the Snowy Range sparkle in the starlight.

"Why economics?" I asked. I knew essentially nothing about the "dismal science."

"I was a math major at the University of Maine in Presque Isle."

I raised my eyebrows, knowing he grew up in Colorado and South Texas. He explained that when he was ready for college, he wanted snow and winter, so he drove north into Canada, then circled back across the border and came to Presque Isle, the farthest-north college town in Maine. One of his math professors there gave him a copy of E. F. Schumacher's book *Small Is Beautiful.*

"What Schumacher said made sense to me. I thought economics could make the world a better place. I imagined using its analysis tools to help us make better decisions for the planet."

After he married Molly's mother, they moved to Pennsylvania for Richard's master's degree and Molly was born. When Richard applied to PhD programs, he was offered assistantships at two schools: the University of Michigan and the University of Wyoming. The former was more prestigious; the latter promised interesting research in valuing natural resources, like clean air and open space. "So, we moved to Laramie." *Of course.* I already knew that intellectual challenge, not status, motivated Richard.

He smiled. "How else would we have met?" He leaned over for a long, slow kiss.

The morning after we saw the circular outline in his MRI images, we ate breakfast in a familiar coffeehouse in Boulder. I wrote in my journal; Richard read *Thinking with Things*, an anthropologist's look at what we say with forms and images. He had told me earlier that the book, a gift from my editor, was helping him understand why he was drawn to abstract sculpture and, in particular, to working with native rocks.

"What are you learning?" I asked.

"I can't articulate it yet, but I'm seeing new ideas for sculptures."

Richard's cell phone buzzed. It was Brooke, reporting that Neurosurgery had a Friday opening ten days hence. If we could make it, Richard would be admitted to the hospital the afternoon before for tests; Neurosurgery would do the biopsy the next day.

"You could go home as early as Saturday," Brooke said.

Richard looked at me for confirmation. *We don't have time for this*, I thought, suddenly panicky. *I have feature article deadlines, teaching, book events. He has two sculpture commissions. Friends from out of town are arriving soon. . . ..* I took a deep breath. *It's just a biopsy*, I reminded myself. *Data. They'll put a needle into his brain and suck out some tissue, and we'll learn something.* I nodded my assent.

I simply couldn't allow myself to imagine anything seriously wrong. When we face the worst, our fears can paralyze us in denial, where I was. The birds were long gone, and the brain swelling had subsided; Richard was his robust self. All had to be well.

Later, while I went to a meeting, Richard sat outside in the fall sunshine and wrote in his journal:

*I thought about the series I started with 4 x 4s [granite river rocks sawed into four-by-four-inch blocks] for the Art Walk auction. They were simple, relatively: a reversal of convexity & smoothness, & I was exploring things I could do at the boundary between convex-rough/concave-smooth.*

*I'd like to do more in this series. I see possibilities to be playful. I'd like to do a cube with one face left convex-rough but for a concave smooth reversal polished in the middle, with all other faces left rough-sawn. . . .. Or the inside could be hollowed out so the whole thing is a lid. The rock might be too small to make a cube, so the cube shape could be completed by extending the 4 sawn sides down with steel. The steel could be galvanized, polished, patinated, painted . . .*

When we left the city, Richard took the wheel. The highway wound up rock-muscled mountain slopes, through pine and fir forests freckled with shrubs in autumn orange, yellow, gold, burgundy, and the occasional scarlet.

We watched for wildlife, continuing our good-natured competition to score the wild ungulate quadrifecta, a game we had invented to enliven the now-too-familiar drive to Denver. The prize went to the one who spotted the most species. Mule deer were the most common, elk and pronghorn next-most likely, and bighorn sheep the most difficult to see. Spotting two species counted as a duofecta; three, a trifecta; the rare times when we spotted all four equaled a quadrifecta. That day, I won with a trifecta of deer, elk, and pronghorn.

Two-plus hours later, winding down Trout Creek Pass into our own valley, Richard slowed the car. "Let's take a detour." Turning onto a gravel road through grassland studded by patches of aspen and piñon pines, he stopped to explore promising rock outcrops, filling the back of the car with slim basalt columns he imagined using for the legs of sculptural tables. I shot photos of golden aspen leaves and sumac in hunter orange. Richard whistled at a chickadee. Life felt normal again.

"Normal" is a hypothetical construct, not reality. It's what we expect or hope to happen—like people being more civil and less hateful, or the oceans not heating up. It's the familiar we crave. Normal is self-defined, a fiction that our minds edit to suit our preferred narrative. When life throws us out of "normal," we long for its comfort. Whichever story we prefer.

By the time we reached Olympia on our honeymoon trip, Richard's tumor had permanently altered our lives. What had become normal would have been unimaginable to the couple exploring rocks and brilliant fall foliage on that sun-warmed Colorado afternoon.

*ghostly circle*
*haunts your right brain*
*your hands still speak rock*

# chapter seven

❧

## Day Eight

### Odometer Reading: 1,461 Miles

At the Sunday-afternoon Tweit clan gathering at Bill and Lucy's, we all pretended Richard was normal. No one mentioned the words "brain cancer," asked about his moon face, or noted his protuberant eyes and paunch. Even the Zipper, Richard's name for the reverse question mark–shaped brain-surgery scar that scribed the right side of his shaved head from stem to stern, attracted no questions, except from the youngest kids, our great-nieces and nephews, who were at the age where that ropy pink ridge was gruesome and thus fascinating.

"Does it hurt?" Fiona, the eldest of the four younger kids, and thus the ringleader, asked. She eyed her great-uncle with her head cocked, a hand on one hip, and her brown hair tossed to one side. Her younger brother looked on, eyes wide.

"Not anymore." Richard bent forward in his seat. "You can touch it if you want."

Fiona and Bubba reached up. "Gently!" cautioned their mom, my middle niece, Sienna, aware that under it lay a titanium plate covering the hole sawed through his skull.

As I aimed the car toward the coast the next morning, I wondered if Richard realized how much brain cancer treatment had altered his appearance. Probably not—our self-image stems more from memory than from mirror. Who we think we are may be years or even decades behind who we have become. It's what keeps us feeling young, but it can also get us into trouble.

The cognitive and emotional impairments resulting from repeated scalpel sculpting of his brain, plus two years of cancer treatment, did get Richard into trouble. He got cheerfully lost even on streets he'd walked for decades—I no longer let him explore on his own. He sometimes got frustrated deciphering his laptop screen; maps and cell phone keypads could be equally baffling. Each morning, we wrote a list on one of the index cards he kept in his shirt pocket so he could remember his plans for that day. I had accepted Richard's impairments, although I wasn't inured to them. For others, the changes were shocking, distressing, even scary.

We have narrowed our definition of what is "normal" to the point that we exclude anyone who is different, whether physically, mentally, or culturally. Those outside the arbitrary lines we draw become targets of revulsion, fear, or bullying. It's as if they are no longer human. I don't know that Richard noticed when people shrank from him. I noticed, and I hurt for him.

That afternoon, we stopped in Seaside, Oregon, to visit the poet David Lee and his wife, Jan. As we parked, Dave called out a booming welcome from the door, Jan smiling next to him. Their smiles faded as Richard lurched up the walk, his gait unsteady. I wanted to say something comforting, to remind us all that the impaired Richard they saw was still the same brilliant and funny person inside, but that wasn't entirely true, and I didn't want to embarrass Richard.

After a shocked moment, Dave turned up the Texas-heartiness in his greeting and launched into a story. No one addressed the elephant. We all pretended.

Back on Highway 101 later, as we headed south toward Waldport for the night, Richard said, "It was great to see Dave and Jan." His voice was sad. "But it's exhausting."

"Trying to be the pre–brain surgery Richard?" I reached for his hand.

He nodded, picked up a beach pebble he'd found at our lunch stop, and closed his eyes. He was asleep, rock in hand, before I reached cruising speed.

A memory popped into my mind, from a hot afternoon in southern Arizona some twenty years before. We had stopped at a rest area on the way home from visiting Mom and Dad in Tucson. When I returned from the bathroom, Richard and Molly were not at the car.

"Suz!"

I looked up. Richard was balanced on a volcanic boulder ten feet above me, leading Molly, then a long-limbed twelve-year-old, on a free climb. They spidered up the rock, defying gravity. I held my breath until they were safely back on the ground.

His body still recognized rocks.

On Friday night of the hospital stay for what we thought was a biopsy, Richard was explaining his ideas for a series of wall sculptures using rounded rocks from the Arkansas River, near our house, when Dr. Ho, whose tan face and dark eyes reminded me of sunny Hawaii, arrived for the surgery-consent process. The neurosurgery team, he told us, had decided on brain surgery, instead of a simple biopsy: "That way, if it's a tumor, we can remove it on the spot."

Shocked into silence by the picture of their cutting open Richard's skull, I listened to Dr. Ho's calm recitation of the risks, including paralysis, blindness, loss of speech and memory, and death. I was not prepared—for brain surgery or the possibility of Richard's death.

I had thought about my own. When I was twenty-three and struggling with a severe relapse of lupus, death was in my forecast. As I learned how to manage the most debilitating symptoms, my focus shifted to life, challenges and all. I started to take better care of myself, and thus improved even more, which motivated me to continue paying attention and practicing self-care.

The sneaky thing about living in a more aware, self-nurturing way is that we actually can become healthier and outlive the estimates. I had no way of knowing then that what I learned about living mindfully in the shadow of death, especially the "fully" part, would turn out to be just the wisdom Richard and I needed—for his death, not mine.

The flashing light of my cell phone signaling a call woke me in the darkness the next morning. I answered groggily, expecting Richard's voice. Instead, it was Tracy, the night nurse at my folks' complex, calling to say that Mom had just been "transported" to the emergency room. "She's not in danger, but her breathing is impaired and she's dizzy."

*Hell.* I dressed hurriedly and called Dad as I navigated across the city. He reported that Mom was "fine" and they were waiting for test results.

"Can you come keep me company?" Mom asked. "I don't like it here."

My stomach clenched. "Mom, Richard is scheduled for brain surgery this morning."

"That's today?" Her voice was surprised. "How is he?"

"It's still early, Mom. I haven't seen him yet."

"Tell him we love him," she said, sounding more like herself.

When I was a kid, Mom was my hero. I was small—I'm the blonde with the Dutch-boy haircut sitting cross-legged in the front row of my first-grade class picture. Mom taught me how to stand up for myself and gave me the gift of reading and nature, my refuges. Despite being color-blind—Mom saw the world in shades of gray through thick-lensed glasses—she was a voracious reader who earned a master's degree in library science. She also organized and led our family outings. On backpacking trips, she headed up the trail with sure steps, our bedrolls lashed to her creaking pack frame. Dad followed, carrying our meals, plus our camp stove and tents; my brother and I trailed, toting jackets and snacks. Mom's voice lulled us to sleep, telling the stories of the constellations; she sang us awake, perfect pitch giving her a thrush's fluting clarity. She loved wildflowers and birdsong, mountain peaks, and all of life.

By the time Richard saw birds, however, Mom's light had dimmed from decades of living with severe rheumatoid arthritis. I worried as her frame shrank from a sturdy five foot six to a petite five two and her weight dropped below ninety pounds. Yet when I expressed concern, she who had helped me learn to manage my health seemed curiously detached from her own. "I'm fine, Suz," she'd say. "Don't fuss."

"I'm fine" could be the motto of my Norwegian-Swedish-Scots heritage. We're stoic, proud, and stubbornly independent sorts who cope first, and if we collapse, we do it in private—after we have taken care of the crisis. That kind of response is a classically female one, emblematic of us as caregivers to the world: *I'll just push through this, and then everything will be fine.* Only one crisis blends into the next and the next. Eventually, we do crash. I hadn't. Yet.

A hundred winding coastal miles and four hours after our visit with Dave and Jan, we turned off at Beverly Beach State Park for a pee break. (Richard had managed a whole day without accidents—a trip record.) Knots of people streamed under the highway overpass toward the beach. I was puzzled, and then realized: the sunset! I dashed to the car for my camera, and we followed the chattering throng just as the shimmering orange ball touched the ocean. As the crowd hushed, Richard took my hand. We stood silent with the others while the sun slipped below the horizon and vanished. Then, as if a switch had flipped, people began talking and laughing again.

Road trip rule number six: Pay attention.

I was breathing hard from climbing five flights of stairs by the time I entered Richard's room that morning of his first brain surgery. *He looks great*, I thought—until he turned his head.

The right side of his shaved skull was studded with marble-size green balls cupped in white plastic bases, each circled in black ink: markers to guide the surgeons as they cut through scalp, muscle, bone, and membrane to reveal his brain. My stomach clenched and rolled.

Richard saw me and smiled. I swallowed, crossed the room, and hugged him. I recounted the call from Tracy and the conversation with Mom.

"Remember when we came to town for my second MRI?" he asked.

That time, Mom had gone to the hospital with pneumonia. "It feels like whenever my attention is diverted, she has a health crisis," I said. "I don't know how long I can handle this." I knew I sounded whiny, but I couldn't help it.

Richard pulled me into his arms. "Once I'm past this surgery, I can help again." I nodded against his chest. I longed for normal, for simply living.

A few minutes later, Richard's neurosurgeon, Dr. Brega, chic even in surgery scrubs, knocked on the open door and walked in. She smiled, told Richard he looked great, and began explaining the process: In the operating room, they would secure his head in place with metal pins. "We don't want your head moving during a craniotomy," she added, with a small grin.

I shuddered at the image of Richard pinned like an insect in a specimen case.

Once the surgeons could "take a look" at what showed up as a circle in the MRI, according to Dr. Brega, if it was indeed a tumor, they would carefully cut it out.

"We don't take any more tissue than we need to." The grin flickered across her face again. "You need all of your brain, so we're pretty conservative."

Richard mentioned that I might have to leave to pick up my parents from another hospital while he was in surgery. Dr. Brega looked sympathetic. "I'll make sure the OR nurse has your cell phone number," she said. Then she headed off to "gather" her team.

At nine thirty, an aide arrived with a rolling bed to take Richard to pre-op. She was startled but delighted when he stood up and asked to walk. I hugged him, and then off my love strode down the hall, head jewelry and all, beside the aide and the unnecessary bed. I heard the aide chuckle when Richard, ever the gentleman, opened the door for her, something I suppose most patients headed for brain surgery aren't in any position to think of, much less do.

By 2:20 that afternoon, Mom and Dad were home and recovering. I fidgeted in my seat in the crowded surgery waiting room, silently reciting my Richard mantra: *May Richard be healthy. May Richard be whole. May Richard be happy and well . . .*

When Dr. Brega and Dr. Ho appeared at the door about forty-five minutes later, I jumped up.

Dr. Brega smiled. "Richard is talking, he can move all of his limbs, and his vision seems normal." She pulled off her surgical mask and brushed chin-length blond hair from her face.

"It was indeed a tumor." Her tone was as satisfied as if she were announcing the sex of a baby. "It was shaped like a marble, seemed to be intact, and was well differentiated from the surrounding tissue."

"A marble?" I focused on the one thing my mind could grasp. "How big?"

She formed her thumb and forefinger into a circle roughly the size of a shooter marble. "It was purple." Dr. Ho nodded in agreement.

"A purple marble." I opened my laptop. "I have to show you his latest sculpture."

I clicked on a photo of *Matriculation*, which Richard had installed in a public sculpture garden that July, before the birds. Dr. Brega and Dr. Ho leaned in to look. Two chiseled blocks of three-foot-high gray volcanic building stone stood open like the covers of a giant book; atop them, a longer and narrower stone perched like a slanting lintel, studded with 128 marbles.

"Good thing he wasn't working with bowling balls," Dr. Brega said drily.

The three of us cracked up. "Great sculpture," Dr. Ho said.

Dr. Brega smiled warmly. "Richard did well."

"Thanks to you and the whole team." My voice wavered. "I surely do love that guy."

Dr. Brega patted my shoulder, and then the two of them headed down the hall. I called my parents to share the good news, and then Molly and my brother.

When the ICU nurse fetched me to Richard's room an hour later, I barely recognized the man I loved. The right side of his shapely head was grossly swollen. A blood-crusted incision—the Zipper—closed with shiny metal staples, ran from his forehead to the back of his head, and then forward and down in front of his right ear. One eye was black. Three bloody holes in his scalp marked where the pins had bitten into his skin. Electrodes sprouted from his chest and upper arms, an oxygen tube chuffed into his nose, and an arterial line snaked from his left forearm.

I felt dizzy but forced a smile. "There's my love." I reached for his hand and sat down quickly, before I passed out.

"I feel like I've been run over by a truck." His voice was hoarse and too loud.

"You've had brain surgery. But you're going to be okay. You can see and talk; you recognized me."

He squeezed my hand and tried to smile. "I'm glad to see you."

Then misery set in: His neck spasmed from being cranked at an awkward angle through four hours of surgery; his head hurt from the incision and skull plate. (At least his brain didn't hurt—brains, which process our bodies' pain signals, feel no pain themselves.) The nurse ordered more pain meds. I held his hand, transmitting comfort. By the time he fell asleep, it was dark. Sleet rattled the window outside, as if winter had come early.

On night eight of our honeymoon trip, the full moon rose, butter yellow, over the Yaquina River as we stopped for dinner in Newport, Oregon. I parked at the old Rogue Ales Pub on the waterfront. Inside the crowded space, a sign on the wall over the bar caught my eye:

DARE *** RISK *** DREAM

I read it to Richard. "That could be the motto for our trip."

"It's a good way to live."

"That's how you've been living," I said. "And why you have inspired so many people."

His eyes teared up, and I heard my use of the past tense. As if he were gone already. "And you are still inspiring people," I amended quickly.

"Thank you," he said, then took a long drink of his porter.

*we dream and dare*
*the way salmon swim out to sea*
*moon their only light*

# chapter eight

*Day Nine*

Odometer Reading: 1,758 Miles

"He's so inspiring." The woman settled a sleek purple bike helmet over silver curls. "Is this really your honeymoon?"

I nodded. "Yes, about twenty-nine years late."

"You're lucky to have each other."

I hadn't felt lucky the night before, as I lugged our gear up the stairs to the motel room and found Richard standing helpless at the door, unable to figure out how to open it. By the time I shepherded him through medications, tooth brushing, and undressing, I was cranky. He fell asleep while I lay awake, bleary-eyed and wondering again how we would manage.

After waking to the deep hoot of the foghorn and a world as gray as I felt, we wound our way down-coast into sunshine. Yellow evening primroses flooded the roadsides; my smile returned. We stopped at the Green Salmon Coffeehouse in Yachats, ordered pastries and hot drinks, and found seats among a crowd biking the coast highway. Richard chatted with the woman next to us; I opened my laptop to write in my journal.

"We are lucky." I replied. And didn't say, *For however long "we" last.*


We went into Richard's first brain surgery dreadfully naive. Neither of us had ever had surgery before, much less lost a chunk of brain, and neither of us took medications regularly. We had no idea how much the drugs and surgery would impact him and, thus, our lives.

Everything went smoothly at first. By Saturday afternoon, just twenty-four hours after his craniotomy, Richard had passed all of the benchmarks for physical and cognitive recovery, impressing his team. That evening, his ICU nurse helped me transfer him to the regular ward. By the following Monday, he was released to go home, less than three days after brain-altering surgery.

It didn't occur to me that Richard's ability to walk around the hospital ward while carrying on an intelligent conversation, which so impressed Phil, the physical therapist, was a long way from actual recovery. A craniotomy is like a brain injury, Dr. Brega said later. It might take a year for the brain to heal entirely, and almost as long for the anesthesia to dissipate. His brain didn't get that recovery time: The second craniotomy came ten months later, the third and fourth a mere five months after that.

When I drove Richard away from the hospital that October Monday, I was just relieved to be heading home. We stopped to visit my parents, who were delighted to see him seeming like his old self but for the sinuous scar scribing the right side of his handsome head.

At home, I imagined settling back into a quiet routine with Richard napping, sketching sculpture ideas, and reading in the comfort of his favorite chair as he recovered. Only the guy who had always prided himself on being calm and unflappable was now everything but, his moods reversing in an instant from cheerful and smiling to snappish, followed by black silence. I learned to be cautious, test the air, and choose my words carefully.

Friday morning, four days after returning home, as he ate breakfast, I said, "I need to finish the draft of the *Audubon* magazine article. Can you give me two hours undisturbed?"

"That's reasonable," upbeat Richard replied. But by the time I settled in to write, distracted and depressed Richard popped into my office every few minutes for reassurance.

Before long, my patience ran out. "Go meditate!" I snapped. "You promised not to interrupt me and promised to resume your practice. You haven't done either. Meditation will help you focus and stop feeling sorry for yourself."

As soon as the words left my mouth, I regretted them—too late.

Richard lunged at me, face enraged, hands raised to strike. My heart raced. He out-matched me by six inches and sixty-five pounds. But my brain was uninjured; I could think more quickly.

I slipped around him and outside, racing along the porch, past his studio, and down the alley, shaking. I looked over my shoulder before dropping out of sight behind my thinking rock, a chest freezer–size boulder perched on the creek bank next to a sagebrush shrub I had planted as a seedling a decade before.

Huddled on the cold ground, back against granite, I breathed in the sweet rosin of sagebrush leaves as tears coursed down my cheeks. I had thought I knew Richard's temper: slow to provoke, words keen as a blade. He might sulk for days, but would never threaten me. (I'm a redhead: I go off like a rocket, all flash and noise. But when it's over, it's over.) A memory surfaced:

Richard pulled our truck up to the condo complex where Molly's mother lived, and I spotted eight-year-old Molly sitting on the split-rail fence, watching the road. I wondered how long she'd been waiting there. She leaped up and ran over on long, colt-like legs. Richard jumped down and swung her into his arms. They cried and laughed and talked at the same time. "You're here!" "I've missed you so much!" He twirled Molly around until they collapsed, laughing, in the grass.

The Richard who was overjoyed to see Molly after a month apart would never threaten me. This Richard? I wasn't sure. I hugged my arms around my knees and tried to think.

Before I found an answer, I began shivering. Time to go back.

Richard met me at the door, arms open, offering a hug. I evaded, then turned to face him, determined. "You threatened me. You were enraged."

"I didn't feel angry," he said. "Or I didn't notice it."

My entire body tensed. "That last statement doesn't make me feel safer."

He reached for my hand, face contrite. "I'm sorry, Suz. I truly didn't mean to scare you."

I drew a deep breath. "You did. And I don't seem to have gotten past the mad."

"Can't we sit together on the couch? We don't have to talk."

"Give me time to simmer down first."

He started to protest. I interrupted with a firmness I rarely used. "Give me ten minutes." I stalked into my office. I sat at my computer but couldn't write. I was still angry, but not, I realized, at Richard—I was furious and frightened by the sudden shift in our lives. He needed me in ways neither of us had imagined. And his surgery-altered brain couldn't grasp the changes.

One of the ironies of caregiving is that we who give the care face the delicate and difficult task of tending a person who is no longer who they think they are. Crises alter us in ways we cannot see, and our self-image is slow to adjust. Or never does. Caregivers—we who are on the first line of defense—take the brunt of those changes. Another irony is in the origin of the word "care" itself: It comes from a German root related to "grieve" or "lament," and from a Norse word meaning "sickbed." We who care tend the sickbed, whether a person, a community, or our planet. And we also grieve the inevitable losses.

Later, Richard admitted that waiting for the pathology results on his tumor had him on edge. I asked what would help him deal with the stress, my words sounding to my ears more like those of a counselor than a lover. He thought. "I'll resume sitting for meditation each morning. And I'll write in my journal. Juggling would help, too: It feels good to coordinate brain and hand."

This time he followed through, and his moods leveled out some. Talking with his neurology and neurosurgery teams about the effects of the surgery and medications helped me.


Until his second craniotomy, ten months later. As with the first, Richard was determined to be discharged from the hospital on Monday, three days postsurgery. I argued for more time to recover: This surgery had gone deeper, removing most of his right temporal lobe. He brushed aside my concerns, passed the tests easily, and was discharged Monday afternoon. Molly, who had flown in from San Francisco, drove us home. Richard went straight to bed when we got there; Molly and I talked for a while and then hugged good night. I fell asleep right away.

The red numerals of the bedside clock read 1:45 when I woke suddenly. Richard grabbed my shoulders and shook me—hard; my jaws cracked together. "Don't strap me down!" he shouted. His hands slid to my neck and squeezed, those long fingers a vice.

"It's me, sweetie." My voice squeaked, starved for air. "You're home with me."

"Suz?" His voice was groggy. His hands slowly relaxed. "I was having a bad dream."

I gulped a breath and swallowed tears. "It's okay. You're home."

"I love you," he said, and fell asleep again. I paced the dark house, shaking. What if I couldn't talk him down next time?

At the hospital, there was a twenty-four-hour, trained staff; at home, it was just me. And Molly, but I was reluctant to wake her. She would worry, and her daddy would be embarrassed. When I returned to bed, I lay awake, assuring myself that Richard would recover and be himself again. All would be well.

A few days later, Richard's oncologist called to check on him. Richard was out on the front porch, sipping coffee and watching hummingbirds zip from wildflower to wildflower in our native-prairie front yard. I answered and poured out the story of our first night at home.

"Did he hurt you?" Dr. Klein's voice was tight.

"No, but he really scared me."

"Don't try to be a hero: call nine-one-one next time. He's bigger and stronger than you are, and the anesthetics and steroids lower his impulse control. As does losing his temporal lobe."

She asked if I had talked to Richard about the incident. I confessed I hadn't. I was worried he'd be angry with himself, and that that might impair his recovery.

She thought a moment. "Worrying about it could set him back. Still, next time, ask for help," she said. "And call me if you need to talk—anytime."

My eyes filled with tears. "Thanks. I'll do that."

The tumors I fervently hoped Richard would survive—I couldn't then imagine life without him—had already altered the landscape of our relationship. He was absorbed in coping with trauma to his brain I couldn't know; I was responsible for us in a way he was no longer capable of understanding. The normal I longed for truly was a fiction.

Thirteen months and three brain surgeries later, we stopped at Devil's Churn Wayside on the Oregon coast on the ninth day of our belated honeymoon trip. I kept an eye on Richard. Until I stopped to shoot a photo of shiny salal leaves.

I looked up to see Richard walk around the guardrail, heading for the cliff edge. Shit! I raced across spray-slicked rocks and used strength I didn't know I possessed to yank him back.

"Did I scare you?" He looked at my face, which was surely dead white. "I just wanted to see the blowhole up close."

I couldn't speak. As I marched him back, a wave crashed over the spot where he had just stood. People were gathered at the rail, eyes wide.

As we passed through, a woman asked, "Is he okay?"

Richard looked confused. "He's had brain surgery," I said. "He didn't grasp the danger."

I had looked away for only a moment. That was long enough, it seemed, for his altered brain to get his body in trouble. What if I hadn't looked back in time? Caregiving is a daily exercise in making miracles happen.

Later that morning, we stopped near Lincoln City to stroll a boardwalk through a swamp crowded with one of my favorite plants, the cobra lily. These unapologetically carnivorous beings sport leaves modified into insect traps: foot-high vertical tubes topped by a bulbous "head" like a cobra rearing, leafy fangs and all. Cobra lilies are communal hunters: They obtain nitrogen lacking in the waterlogged soils where they live by growing in masses that lure flies, bees, and ants inside those light-filled tubes. Trapped, the insects eventually drown in the pool at the base and microorganisms digest them, liberating their nitrogen and other nutrients, the way the microbes in our guts digest our food. Cobra lilies remind me that life is endlessly creative in its drive to thrive, and that community is critical.

Richard took my hand as we stopped to admire the mass of chartreuse-green tubes, cobra hoods up, as if dancing for an invisible snake charmer. A grin transformed his round face. Just then, a cobalt-blue Stellar's jay landed nearby and chattered.

"I see you, Stellar's jay," Richard said. "But right now I'm admiring the cobra lilies."

Two hours and a hundred winding miles later, we visited historian and author Ann Vileisis and her husband, photographer Tim Palmer, in their home at Port Orford. Ann and I knew each other through our respective writing but had never met. When she heard about the Big Trip, she invited us to stop by. Richard sparkled, his smile and conversation bright, as Ann and Tim showed us their house, a renovated church with walls lined with books, and their flower-filled garden, buzzing with pollinators.

When we hugged goodbye, Ann whispered into my ear, "Thanks for sharing Richard. He's a gift."

I was surprised and then realized: They didn't know the old Richard. They simply appreciated the extraordinary man now, brain damage and all.

"Thank you for reminding me," I said, humbled and teary.

*steps shaky*
*you reach for my hand*
*love smooths this trail*

# chapter nine

❦

## Day Ten

### Odometer Reading: 2,005 Miles

On the morning of our tenth day on the road, we wandered hand in hand in awed silence through a grove of coast redwoods in Northern California, our footsteps muffled by the deep mantle of fallen needles. Shafts of sunlight slipped between the trunks of trees taller than most skyscrapers and older than Western civilization; the fluting songs of hermit thrushes echoed around us.

What makes redwood groves so humbling is more than the staggering size and age of the trees. Tree-climbing scientists have discovered hundreds of species inhabiting their arboreal forms, from marbled murrelets—robin-size, oceangoing seabirds that nest on branches thirty stories up—to banana slugs on the ground, grazing on lichens blown from high above. In between, entire metropolises, millions of individuals, interweave their lives. No wonder these groves feel holy—they are living cathedrals honoring the abundance and diversity of life itself.

Richard stopped to admire a redwood so tall its top was out of sight. As he turned toward me, my camera captured the smile lighting his face, his arms raised in utter joy.

I heard again his question from the first night of the trip: "Why didn't we do this sooner?"

Why didn't we take more time to slow down? Pursue our ter-raphilia? The usual reasons: It is human nature to get caught up in daily demands: raising families, working, paying bills, cooking, cheering our teams, tending elderly parents . . . We rarely stop to consider why the rush, what our lives mean. We forget to value happiness. Joy. Until some jolt reminds us that life is finite. And living with love—for each other and for this planet—is what lasts.

For us that jolt came a week after Richard's first brain surgery, when we headed to Denver for his postsurgery checkup. We met with Brooke Allen first. After commenting about how great Richard looked, she asked if he was tolerating the drugs. "Have you had any crankiness?"

"No."

His response was so confident that I almost choked. Brooke turned to me, eyebrows raised.

"He has no patience." I looked at Richard. "I'm sorry, sweetie, but it's true. You've always been known for your even-tempered-ness, but not now."

I added that Richard, who never cussed—unlike me—now used the f-word frequently. I didn't mention his rage. That was tender still. I did say, "I wonder if he should be driving."

"No," Brooke's voice was as sure as Richard's response had been. "No driving until you're off the antiseizure medications."

He looked at me, eyes accusing, as if I had betrayed him. "I think of myself as calm and peaceful, because that's how I feel inside."

"You are even-tempered, Richard," Brooke said. "But you're taking two medications known to depress impulse control and raise aggressive tendencies. This behavior isn't you, it's the drugs. You both need to stay aware and be patient. You love each other. That will help."

I leaned over and gave Richard an apologetic kiss. He squeezed my hand.

Then came Neurosurgery, where Dr. Brega reported the pathology results: brain cancer.

Fifteen thousand Americans die of brain cancer each year, the majority of them men between the ages of forty and seventy. The cause of primary brain cancer—tumors like Richard's, which begin in the brain, rather than elsewhere in the body—is still a mystery. Cancer comes in many flavors, but all result from ordinary genetic mutations that alter a cell's behavior, allowing it to divide without limits and avoid normal apoptosis, cell death. Death is healthy; the "undead" cells continue dividing unchecked, crowding out healthy tissue. The causes of the mutation and the trigger that turns on that damaged genetic switch are as varied as the kinds of cancers and their outcomes. The prognosis of glioblastoma, the type of brain tumor Richard had, is grim: a few months to a decade, with a median of 14.6 months. He lived twice that long.

The word itself had ironic significance for us: Cancer is the name of the small, crab-shaped constellation that is Richard's sign in the zodiac; thus, in astrology, he was born into cancer.

After hearing that diagnosis from Dr. Brega, we walked down the stairs in silence and out to the parking garage. I drove. Richard didn't argue. We stopped to visit my parents but didn't mention cancer. We were still in shock.

Less than a week later, we set out on a two-week road trip to New Mexico and Texas for events I had scheduled months earlier—before the birds—to promote my new book. We needed time away from brain cancer and parent care—time together to simply live.

The night before we left, I woke from a vivid dream, heart pounding. Mom called from the hospital. "I need you. Please come." Her voice was thin and shaky, terrified. Lying on my back in the darkness, Richard breathing evenly next to me, I reminded myself that Mom was fine. She had Dad. And I needed a break.

The previous winter, I realized Mom had lost interest in cooking, and even in eating regularly (unless I prepared the meals). I suggested she and Dad consider moving to a retirement complex with a meal plan. They were fine, they insisted. A month later, Mom announced suddenly that they had decided to move to a place that provided meals. "You'll help find us the right place," she said. We did, and supervised their move, too.

Caring for aging parents means assuming a quasiparental role, only without parental authority. It's like dealing with teenagers whose brains have not matured along with their bodies. Sometimes our parents are happy to let us take the lead, and they even follow our suggestions. Other times, they respond with the equivalent of the raised middle finger, reminding us with haughty dignity or outright anger that they are still in full control of their lives. Yet we caregiving kids are responsible when things go wrong.

Mom loved their new apartment, with its view of cottonwood trees along an irrigation ditch. Her daily emails reported enthusiastically on the dawn bird chorus, walks to nearby parks, bus tours to the mountains for picnics, and meals in the dining room. She gained ten pounds. And then, gradually, she began to slip again. Her blue eyes lost their sparkle, and her smile appeared less often. She seemed more forgetful and needy, less engaged in the world.

After we loaded the car, Richard tucked his briefcase behind the driver's seat and said, "I want to drive." I thought about Brooke Allen's prohibition and weighed it against the benefits of Richard at the wheel: Driving was something he enjoyed, and it would help him feel in control, rather than helpless. Both of those factors might alleviate his still-touchy moods. I slipped into the passenger seat.

As he drove us south on snowy roads, Richard commented that our route to Austin would roughly parallel the one he took when he left Texas at age seventeen, in 1968, headed for his childhood home in Colorado.

A photo of that Richard on my desk showed a tall, sinewy young man leaning against a brick wall, right leg folded under him, balancing the guitar he strummed. The sleeves of his plaid button-down shirt were rolled up; his jeans were trendy white. Straight, dark hair flopped over a high forehead; dark brows lined somber eyes gazing off to the side—a young, troubled James Dean. I wanted to fold that boy into a hug, make him laugh, and love the sadness away.

I knew little about the summer that had caused a rift between Richard and his family. I also knew an oblique approach would be more successful in eliciting that story than a direct one. "What was Austin like then?" I asked.

It was the height of the Vietnam War, Richard reminded me, and he was a country boy fresh out of high school. His draft number was low; his eighteenth birthday loomed.

"I had no idea what I wanted from life. I only knew I didn't believe in the war and couldn't in good conscience go to college just to get a deferment."

He found a job with the University of Texas grounds crew. While laying sod, he watched ambulances scream by, bound for a nearby trauma hospital, and realized that he wanted to save lives, not end them.

"I decided to apply for conscientious-objector status, only I didn't know how."

(In an odd bit of synchrony, I began attending Quaker meetings that same summer, drawn by Friends' support of conscientious objectors and opposition to the war.)

On Richard's next trip home to Eagle Pass, he told me, he called the minister of his church. The minister agreed to meet with Richard and then phoned Richard's father. When Richard arrived at the minister's office in the soft South Texas dusk, his father was waiting outside. Mr. Raymond told his middle son that he would make sure the church did not support him. If Richard pursued conscientious-objector status, Mr. Raymond said, the family would be shamed and Richard would no longer be welcome at home.

Hurt and confused, Richard caught a late-night bus back to Austin, quit his job, and hit the road, guitar and duffel in hand. He hitchhiked across the lonely spaces of West Texas to El Paso, where his circuit-riding, Methodist-preacher grandfather had died of tuberculosis in 1918, just weeks after Richard's father and his twin brother were born. From there, Richard followed the Rio Grande north to Colorado and Salida, where he bought a 1950 Chevy pickup and found work logging in the mountains. He camped with a coworker and recalled playing his guitar by their campfire at night, eating a lot of beans, and reading Helen and Scott Nearing's *Living the Good Life: How to Live Sanely and Simply in a Troubled World.*

Richard's family eventually tracked him down, and he reluctantly agreed to meet them in Sonora, on the edge of the hill country. That tense encounter resulted in a compromise: Richard would enroll in college. After one semester, though, he dropped out and enlisted in the Coast Guard.

"I thought I would be pulling drowning people from the surf," he told me. "I ended up maintaining the communications towers that guided bombers and nuclear submarines to Vietnam."

And drinking to dull the pain of his complicity in the war: "We went through so many cases of liquor every week, our trash cans clinked." After the Coast Guard, Richard returned to Austin and found work in a cabinet shop. A year later, he built a camper for his pickup and headed north, landing in Maine, where he reenrolled in college and met Molly's mother.

As the road miles ticked past, Richard relaxed into his even-tempered self again. We talked about the irony that enlisting in the Coast Guard had made him eligible for VA health care benefits neither of us had expected him ever to need—until the birds.

We also talked about his father, Mr. Raymond, who grew up fatherless, the youngest of seven children in a family that struggled to cling to gentility. "Mr. Raymond loved you," I said. "He must have feared that you, his dreamy middle son, would struggle financially, the way his own family did when he was young."

Richard thought. "Thank you for seeing him so generously. That helps me understand."


In Austin, Richard toured galleries in the steamy heat, sketched sculpture ideas in his notebook, juggled acorns he picked up under the city's historic Treaty Oak tree, and got a traffic ticket. After the courteous motorcycle cop took Richard's license, I could feel my love's temper rise. I reminded him of his nightly intention: "To live with lovingkindness for all."

Richard glared at me. I took his hand. "I love you."

That got through. "Was I worrying you?"

"Yes," I held my ground.

"I don't want to do that. My aim is to be a source of support and joy."

"I know that. But you're still taking the cranky drugs."

When the officer returned, Richard made an effort to be friendly. The patrolman asked what brought us to Austin. Richard offered a copy of his sculpture brochure; I handed him a postcard showing my books. The officer promised to look us up in Colorado sometime.

As he pulled away, Richard turned to me. "Thank you."

"For what?"

"Helping me to live with lovingkindness." He grinned. "Despite the cranky drugs."

Two nights later, as we walked across downtown Austin at dusk after the Texas Book Festival, a bat fluttered across my vision, and then another. I looked up to follow their flight and saw the full moon, huge and golden as a sunset, shimmering through the city haze.

"Look!"

Richard looked up and spotted the moon, and then a third bat, fluttering across the sky, directly in front of that brilliant orb. He beamed. "I'm a lucky guy." He leaned down to kiss me.


A week after returning home, we drove to Denver to meet Richard's oncologist. We arrived in the city the evening before, bearing dinner for my parents, only to find they weren't home. Mom had been "transported" (you've got to love jargon that evokes images of flying carpets) to the hospital for dehydration. We raced there and found her frail-looking but recovering, so we drove Dad home and fed him. Then we headed across the city to Fisher House, housing for out-of-town VA families.

I woke before dawn the next morning, startled by a siren's howl. When I rolled over to stretch aching joints, Richard woke, too. We snuggled sleepily. He looked at the clock.

"It's early. Want to make love?" He pulled me close for a sumptuous kiss.

My mind found plenty of reasons to object, but my body ignored them.


Later, at the waiting room in the VA Medical Center, Richard read *Building a Picture*, a book about abstract sculptor Nathan Slate Joseph, whose "quilts" of recycled metal he had admired in Austin.

"Richard Cabe!" A petite woman with short, tousled hair and a white lab coat stood at the clinic entrance, scanning the crowd. We jumped up and walked over.

She smiled and shook each of our hands firmly. "Catherine Klein. I'm your oncology doctor."

She led us back to her spartan exam room and said to Richard, "I hear you're a sculptor. Tell me about your work."

While he talked, I opened my laptop and showed photos.

Her eyes brightened at the boulder that spouted fire. "I want one of those."

Richard smiled. "That could be arranged."

Then she turned to his treatment plan: six weeks of daily radiation to his right temporal lobe, accompanied by oral chemotherapy. Since the radiation would be administered at the University of Colorado Hospital's cancer center, we would have to move to the city.

I sat silent, stunned. Cancer, uprooter of lives, would wrench us from our quiet home to the noisy city so that Richard's brain could be bombarded with deadly radiation.

"You're relatively young, and you're healthy," Dr. Klein said, "so we want to treat this aggressively. If you were eighty years old, we might not take this course. But you have a good chance of many years of sculpture work ahead."

After our morning with the redwoods, Richard snoozed as I navigated hairpin bends over the Coast Range. When I stopped to shoot a photo of the distant expanse of blue ocean, Richard woke and pointed out a clump of brilliant orange wildflowers. "California poppies!" He took my hand. "Remember the poppies and condors in Big Sur?"

It was February, several years before Richard's birds. We were cruising north up the Big Sur coast to visit Molly, Richard at the wheel. I spotted a blaze-orange swath of California poppies blooming high on a ridge bared by fire the year before. Richard pulled over, and we got out to look. Just then, an enormous, dark bird soared over the ridgetop on wide wings: a California condor, one of the rarest birds in North America. We watched open-mouthed as another condor drifted into view, and another, and another, until seven of them soared on the ocean breeze high overhead.

"I am the luckiest guy in the world," Richard said.

*wild poppies*
*blazing orange and gold*
*stop! look!*

chapter ten

*Day Eleven*

Odometer Reading: 2,224 Miles

Looking across the café table, I saw the scholar I had fallen in love with almost three decades earlier. Richard's face was relaxed, reading glasses perched on his nose, eyes focused on a book on the work of artist-blacksmith Albert Paley. I had no idea if he was still able to make sense of the text or if he was simply "reading" the photos. No matter, he was absorbed, his undamaged left brain as thirsty as ever for knowledge. We sat in a coffeehouse in Fort Bragg, a former lumber-mill town on California's foggy North Coast. Tomorrow we would celebrate my fifty-fifth birthday with Molly in San Francisco. Richard's energy was fading; he often napped while I drove. But his delight in each day, new vista, birdcall, moment was undimmed. He might have been dying, but he was also very much alive.

The trip was both wonderful—literally full of wonder—and painful. And sometimes hilarious, as when the toddler at the next table wandered over, dropped her teething ring on Richard's plate, and grabbed the last bite of his chocolate croissant. Richard laughed and, responding much more quickly than I thought he could, wrestled the pastry out of her sticky hand and slipped the teething ring into the astonished O of her mouth. "No trades," he said with a grin, and popped the squashed chunk of croissant into his mouth.

We sat together every morning like this—he reading, I writing—during the weeks of radiation treatment when we lived in room 6, a sunny, second-floor corner suite at Fisher House in Aurora. As we'd packed for the move, Richard had hauled out his Geek Case, a wide-mouthed leather briefcase that had carried legal briefs in his expert-witness days, and filled it with books: volumes on art theory and abstract sculpture, mindfulness and brain research, and *Anticancer: A New Way of Life*, by David Servan-Schreiber, a physician, neuroscience researcher, and brain-cancer survivor. The book's research-based suggestions on diet and lifestyle supported Richard's program of "extreme health" and gave us hope about living with cancer.

If we were naive about the effects of brain surgery, we were truly unprepared for the way cancer treatment commandeered our lives. When we met Dr. Chen, Richard's radiation oncologist, he informed us in staccato tones that we had wasted too much time already. "No more delays." Richard's radiation treatments, he decreed, *would* begin the Monday after Thanksgiving (at that point, less than two weeks away) and continue through mid-January—"No interruptions. We must attack the cancer now," he said, "before it is too late."

On the drive home over the mountains, we talked about our fears and about our hopes. We vowed to create a positive "radiation residency," like the artist-writer residency we had forgone because of Richard's birds: a regime of contemplative days devoted to reading, writing, and exploring. We were determined to find joy in each day, period.

On our first night in room 6, I finished hanging my clothes in the closet as Richard, seated on the queen-size bed, patted the spread. "We need to test the mattress." His smile was sweet and not at all innocent.

I heard muffled voices from the room next door. "Only if we're really quiet."

"I can be quiet. Can you?"

I laughed. "Probably."

We weren't entirely quiet, but the mattress worked just fine.

Afterward, Richard pulled me close and fell asleep almost immediately, as he invariably did—a skill I envied. I lay awake worrying about our empty house in far-off Salida, about the radiation and chemo, about Richard. The furnace came on with a *whoosh*, a television muttered, a door slammed . . . I drifted off, still worrying.

Each morning, Richard woke in the darkness at four thirty to take his chemo pills on an empty stomach. After he came back to bed, we snuggled and often made love—until the cumulative radiation doses zapped his energy. At six thirty, we rose and did yoga. Then, while Richard showered and shaved, I dressed and padded downstairs to cook our all-organic, whole-grain, high-in-healthy-omega-3-fatty-acids, anticancer, hot breakfast cereal.

After breakfast, we bundled up in jackets, scarves, and caps to walk to a nearby coffeehouse for quiet time. I wrote; Richard read, occasionally sharing bits from the book of the day.

Back at Fisher House, Richard set up his zafu in our walk-in closet and meditated; I sat at the desk and continued writing. At lunchtime, I prepared our meal using whole grains, fruits, and vegetables high in antioxidants and other cancer-fighting compounds and low in the refined sugars and carbohydrates that fuel tumor growth.

I love to cook. It's both fun—a license to play with food and its colors, textures, and flavors—and a way to express love. We are quite literally what we eat. The molecules in our food do more than fuel our metabolism; they are the materials we use to remake our bodies, replacing the continual loss of the proteins that construct our cells. Food nourishes us at many levels. It quiets the physical and mental pangs of hunger and also provides molecular building materials. It stretches our senses through flavor and texture, and it influences our emotions and health via our internal chemistry. Food affects who we become, inside and out, body and soul. I aimed to fill Richard with all the love and goodness healthy food could provide.

After Richard's daily session in "the mask," the molded face mask that immobilized his head while measured doses of gamma rays bombarded his brain, we took a walk around the mile-square medical-school campus. Richard's favorite destination was *Corpus Callosum*, a two-block-long outdoor sculpture by Thomas Sayre named for the channel in our brains that carries information from hemisphere to hemisphere. The steel, granite, and concrete installation stretched between the brick, 1920s Fitzsimons Army Hospital building and the modern, glass-and-steel medical school. Two huge globes anchored the ends: an open sphere of polished steel rods at the modern end; a solid ball of earth-textured, soil-colored concrete at the Army Hospital end. Between them rose a series of upright rectangles of pink granite pierced by round openings; ledges in the openings offered seating with electrical outlets, an allusion to brain wiring.

"What is it that draws you to that particular sculpture?" I asked one night.

Toothbrush in hand, Richard considered my question. "What fascinates me about *Corpus Callosum* is the metaphor. Sayre is using the metaphor of a brain structure that links our two disparate hemispheres with a sculpture linking the old hospital building, state of the art for its era, to the new medical school. He's linking the world of research and teaching to the world of treatment; creativity to intellect; art to science; technology to earth."

"Wow!" I rinsed my mouth. "That's a lot. You should write Sayre with those insights."

Richard nodded and added, "It inspires me to incorporate what I'm learning from living with brain cancer into my own sculpture practice."

*Living with brain cancer. That's all I want*, I thought. *To find a way to be productive and not succumb to grief or anger or fear. To contribute to the light in the world.*


As the days and radiation treatments ticked by, Richard's smile didn't dim, but his energy did. He napped more and read less; we took shorter walks; our lovemaking ceased.

One afternoon, he dozed while I opened the application packet for "33 Ideas," an invitational art show at Denver International Airport named for its thirty-three display cases, each of which would illustrate a different idea. When he had received the invitation to apply, Richard had suggested we collaborate. Then came the birds and brain cancer. Now, I read the call for entries out loud.

"I don't have the energy to come up with an idea," Richard said, face sad.

"Remember how we applied for the Aspen Ridge residency? I wrote a draft, and you added your thoughts. We could use the same process."

His face brightened. "I'd be happy to help. I just can't take the lead right now."

I blinked away sudden tears, and an idea took shape in my mind. "We could invent a word that captures our shared love of the earth and then illustrate the word with our work."

He thought a while and then nodded. "That's promising."

We tossed around words, but none stuck.

At bedtime, Richard said, "'Terraphilia.' Like E. O. Wilson's 'biophilia,' but encompassing the earth itself."

"'Terraphilia' . . ." I tested how the word felt when I said it aloud. "I like it."

The next day, I worked on a definition and statement. We settled on "Terraphilia, n. An intrinsic affection for and connection to the earth and its community of lives. Without this bond we are lonely, lacking, no longer whole." Richard sketched ideas for the showcase. We finished our packet that Friday and hand-delivered it ten minutes before the deadline.

By the third week of our radiation residency, the routine was familiar and Dr. Chen was greeting Richard with a smile and a friendly elbow jab at his weekly check-in.

It was also nearly the winter solstice. At home, we would have been preparing for our annual Light the Darkness party to celebrate the day when the northern hemisphere turns back toward light and spring, toward green and plenty and awakening life. Each year, we invited dozens of friends and family to help line our block with luminarias, small votive candles nested on sand in paper lunch bags, to illuminate winter's longest night. After placing and lighting hundreds of luminarias, the crowd jammed our house to celebrate, sipping gallons of the rich eggnog I made for the occasion.

Richard loved the whole ritual: the luminarias, the eggnog, and the gathering of our community. He was glum about missing the tradition.

"Let's throw a virtual Light the Darkness party," I said one afternoon. "We can invite friends, family, and my readers to light their own luminarias and share photos and celebrations."

Richard smiled for the first time that day. "That's brilliant!"

On the evening of the solstice, I dug out the six white paper bags I had packed, along with candles and a can of sand. As snow fell softly in big flakes, we set our luminarias on the front walk of Fisher House, lit each tiny candle, and stood admiring their glow.

Upstairs in our room, messages winged in from around the country and the world. The taper on a fireplace mantel ("It was raining out, but I didn't want to miss lighting the darkness"), tea lights floating in a pond, luminarias lining the woodland path (which the designer didn't realize before that night was exactly aligned with the setting sun at the winter solstice), luminarias along walls and driveways, patios and courtyards, grouped on a motor-home roof . . . Last came the video showing a crowd of friends gathered at our Salida house to light luminarias and toast Richard's health. Love from around the world lit the real and metaphorical darkness of our longest night.

Richard folded me into his arms. "Thank you," he said.

I mopped streaming eyes. "I'm not the only one who loves you."

Molly arrived a few days later to spend the week between Christmas and New Year's with her daddy while I flew to La Paz, Mexico, to teach a weeklong Writing Adventure workshop on Isla Espíritu Santo, in the Sea of Cortez. I had planned the workshop the year before as a honeymoon trip—the remote desert island in the midst of a subtropical sea was one of our dream destinations. And then came the birds.

After Dr. Chen's decree that Richard's radiation treatments could not be postponed, I had argued for canceling the workshop. I couldn't imagine leaving Richard during that time.

"Sometimes taking care of each other means our paths diverge," Richard reminded me.

I knew he was right, although I hated to admit it. Still, the truth was, I desperately needed a break from cancer and caregiving.

The day after Christmas, Molly and Richard talked animatedly about their plans while driving me to the airport. In the backseat, I reviewed my itinerary, the contents of my rolling duffel, and my fears. So much could go wrong: I was headed to a remote island in Mexico with no cell phone service. My Spanish was less than fluent. I had never led a group abroad, much less solo. And yet something else sprouted through the worry: a tendril of excitement—twined with guilt—about the prospect of a few days of freedom.

When we reached the security checkpoint at the Denver airport, I hugged Molly.

She whispered, "I'll take good care of Dad. Don't worry."

Then Richard pulled me into his arms. "May your trip go smoothly; may you have *fun*."

I blinked back tears. "May you be whole. May you be healthy. May you be happy."

As I walk away, he called, "Don't forget: We share the moon!"

I blew him and Molly a kiss, as much to reassure myself as for them.

To my surprise, all went well once I reached Baja. I relaxed for the first time in months, lulled by the warm sun and birdsong, the lapping of the waves outside our tents on the beach, and the familiar tarry smell of the desert's creosote bush. I watched frigate birds soar high above the tall, many-armed pitaya cacti; listened to the thwacking of brown pelicans diving for fish in the turquoise water; snorkeled with sea lion pups; identified wildflowers; and kayaked with sea turtles. I remembered how much I needed the wild to recharge. To nurture my terraphilia. To help me live with love and compassion.

At the end of that magical week, I spotted Richard and Molly beaming in the crowd beyond security at the Denver airport. We hugged and laughed and talked nonstop. "Next winter, I'll take you both to Isla Espíritu Santo. I can't wait to share it with you."

But by the next winter, my mother was dying. And when Richard and I finally took our belated honeymoon, his right brain was too impaired to travel to an isolated island in Mexico. We decided to drive the Pacific coast instead. That, it turned out, was adventure enough.

> *paseando las olas*
> *el viento canta de peces—*
> *rien*

> *riding the waves*
> *the wind sings of fish—*
> *laughing*

# chapter eleven

## Day Twelve

## Odometer Reading: 2,415 Miles

On Saturday morning in San Francisco, Richard woke cheerful and full of energy—like his old self.

"Let's walk to Caffe Roma. Molly and Mark [her boyfriend] can meet us there."

"We're not at our usual hotel, sweetie. Caffe Roma is a mile away. Let's take a bus."

"We're in San Francisco and it's sunny out," he said. "I feel like walking."

I tried reason, but my guy was determined. Finally, I gave in. Richard strode along confidently, pointing out familiar landmarks—until he tripped and fell headlong, hitting the ground with a sickening *thunk*. I checked him over, heart racing.

"I'm fine." His voice was cranky.

If he was cranky, I thought, he hadn't hurt himself. I helped him up, and on we walked.

A few blocks later, Richard strode right into the traffic on Columbus Avenue.

I yanked him out of the path of a bus. "Don't step into the fucking street without looking!"

"I forgot." His face was contrite. "I was enjoying walking in a city we both love."

My anger evaporated, replaced by shame for yelling at him. I rose on tiptoes and kissed him. "Just stop when you get to a street, okay? I didn't bring you this far to get killed in traffic."

He thought for a moment, considering my request. "That's reasonable," he said, his tone devoid of irony. "Is that rule number seven?"

I choked, caught between laughter and tears.

At the café, Richard debated over the pastries in the glass case before making his choice: a fresh-fig Danish and a chocolate croissant. "Fresh fig would make an interesting Valentine's Day cheesecake," he said with a grin as we settled in to wait for Molly and Mark.

For our first Valentine's Day in 1983, Richard gave me a copy of Mollie Katzen's *The Enchanted Broccoli Cookbook*. Tucked inside was a bookmark cut from pink construction paper on which he wrote, *Hoping this gives you pleasure for a very long time, and hoping we'll share in each other's lives for even longer. With more love than I know how to express, Richard.*

We hadn't known each other two months then, yet already he knew that I love to cook and I cook with love. I reciprocated by making Katzen's amaretto cheesecake, except I didn't have ricotta, so I substituted vanilla yogurt, strained. I couldn't find chocolate wafer cookies in Laramie, either, so I used vanilla wafers crumbled with Dutch cocoa powder. This is how I always cook—and, in fact, how I live: improvising around the recipe the way a jazz musician riffs off a melody. Usually, it works.

That cheesecake did: We made love that night until the air positively glowed.

Cheesecake became our Valentine's Day tradition; each year, I invented a new kind. Richard's favorites included pear-ginger, and dark chocolate marbled with my parents' homemade orange marmalade.

Except for cheesecakes and other special occasions, my cooking in the years Molly was growing up was less focused on being creative than on producing three healthy meals per day for three differing palates. If I was the short-order cook, Richard was the occasional gourmet baker. Molly remembers fondly the from-scratch pot pies he made once, and the Spanish tortilla, a crustless form of quiche he baked for our summer yard parties. I remember the butter croissant he and Molly made one Mother's Day, starting two days in advance and rolling out the papery dough, spreading it with butter, folding, chilling, rolling, and spreading more butter. Those "little crescents" were as flaky and tender as any we ate in France on a winter trip with Molly.

Once we moved into the house he built us in Salida with its generous kitchen, Richard took up bread baking, producing rustic sourdough boules made with whole-wheat flour ground from local grains. Each loaf was an edible sculpture, sensuously round and satisfyingly crusty.

That morning in San Francisco, I tried to recall what flavor cheesecake I had made for Valentine's Day that year. And then I remembered: There had been no cheesecake. Mom had died eleven days before, and Richard was in the VA hospital, recovering from a brain-fluid-accumulation crisis. I vowed I would bake a fig cheesecake for him the next Valentine's Day. I did; he wasn't there to eat it. Seven years passed before I baked another.

After we ate, Richard insisted on walking up the steep hill to Molly and Mark's flat. Our progress was slow, with many stops. Once there, Richard lowered himself into a chair on the deck, with its view of the bay, and closed his eyes. "I think I wore myself out," he said. "San Francisco is a great city for walking, and I wanted to walk across it one more time."

Molly and I looked at each other, tears in our eyes.


I remember a summer day when we were at an overlook on Trail Ridge Road in Rocky Mountain National Park with Molly's grandparents, visiting from Arkansas.

"Suz, look!" Molly's voice turned my attention from the snow-dappled peaks. "I can still do it!"

"It" meant standing on her father's shoulders, as she used to do when she was younger and her legs weren't as long as they were now, at nine. She wobbled in a gust, and my heart stuttered.

Richard put his arms out for balance. "Be a raven and surf the waves," he said. She echoed his movements. They didn't topple. I held my breath until she climbed down, somersaulting nimbly from his chest to the ground for our applause.

*What would I do if I lost them?* I thought, suddenly chilled. And then the even more unthinkable question: *What would they do if they lost each other?*


Once the fatigue from his radiation treatments receded, Richard felt great, until he started monthly oral chemotherapy, a twenty-eight-day cycle he dubbed his "chemo comma," an allusion to the cycle of women's menstrual periods. His comma began with five days of temozolomide, a drug that kills cells by damaging their DNA, followed by twenty-three days to recover, and then a trip to Denver for blood tests. If he passed those, his "reward" was starting over again on the chemo cycle.

Chemotherapy is a war on our own bodies, an expensive and exhausting fight to kill the "bad" cells without harming the "good" ones. When Dr. Klein said that treating brain cancer involved "blunt-force tools," she wasn't kidding. I still wonder if Richard's treatment was worth the time and cost and pain. It didn't save him, but maybe it bought us more time. Perhaps it doesn't matter. What does is that we did our best to find love and joy in each day, grueling or not.

By day five of Richard's first chemo comma, a few days before I would have to leave for a weekend of speaking at back-to-back garden conferences, Richard was miserable. He lay curled up under a blanket in front of the woodstove, shivering with a flu-like fever. And he wasn't eating. The previous night, he had managed only a few bites of his favorite dinner, cheese enchiladas smothered in my special green chile sauce. That morning, in desperation, I offered the Cherry Garcia ice cream he usually couldn't resist.

"I just don't feel like food," he said, his voice weak.

"Are you taking the antinausea medication?" I asked.

"I'm not nauseous," he said, jaw set. "And I'm not taking more medication than I need."

"You're not eating," I responded. "You're shivering and weak. That's what the antinausea meds are supposed to prevent. Don't be so damn stubborn!"

He pulled the blanket over his head. I sat nearby writing and trying not to worry about the road ahead. Not just the drive to Colorado Springs on Friday afternoon for one conference, and on to Fort Collins on Saturday for another, and then back to Denver to move my parents, who had decided to relocate to a smaller apartment one floor up from their current one. Our lives . . .

The next morning, Richard was still weak, but he insisted he was better.

"I want to come with you this weekend. I can be helpful, with the driving, at least."

There was my lever. "Then take the antinausea medication," I said, voice firm. "We'll see how you feel on Friday."

He glared at me. "If you insist, but I don't need it. I'm *not* nauseous."

Caregivers learn to be stubborn and pushy, exercising the muscles of loving courage. Not courage as the word is often used, to mean gritting one's teeth and pushing through, or fighting, but courage in the sense of the word's roots in the old French *corage*, from the Latin for "heart." True courage is strength that comes from the heart—courage that carries the power of love. It takes courage to be honest, to meet with an open heart whatever comes. To practice kindness in a time of hatefulness, to speak truth to power. To live with love in a world awash in fear and grief.

The antinausea medication did the trick; Richard's appetite and energy returned almost immediately. On Friday morning, he unrolled his yoga mat beside mine for the first time in weeks. Over breakfast, he announced, "I'm feeling good. I want to drive."

I watched him savor his hot cereal and fresh-squeezed juice. "Okay."

Driving to Colorado Springs that afternoon, Richard spotted two American dippers, aquatic songbirds, bobbing on rocks in the river. He bobbed his head in time with the motion of the robin-size birds. Eight winding miles later, he stopped so we could watch a herd of five bighorn sheep ewes and two rams as they grazed on new spring grass near the highway. He beamed.

Three days later, we were home again, having successfully navigated both garden conferences and moving my parents to their new apartment. I drank hot chocolate as I answered email; Richard worked a sudoku puzzle and sipped cancer-fighting green tea.

"Here's an email about the Aspen Ridge residency," I said. "The committee voted unanimously to offer us another chance." I looked up. "Want to try for September again?"

Richard looked sad. "I don't know if I could pull any new work together."

"You wouldn't have to. The offer is based on last year's application."

He grinned. "I'll order patina and experiment with sheet metal for wall sculptures."

I grinned back. We *would* be okay.


Thus went that spring—up and down, depending on where he was in the chemo-comma cycle. The downs usually came on day five of the chemo doses. Like the day in March when we drove to Denver to install our terraphilia entry in the "33 Ideas" show. Richard parked in the airport parking garage; opened the back of the car; lifted out *Prosthesis*, his tabletop-size, steel-and-basalt sculpture; and headed for the terminal doors.

I eyed the rest of our materials: satchels of tools and books, banners, and a poster-size photo of his fire-pit sculpture.

"If you wait a minute," I said, "I'll find a luggage cart to haul everything."

"I have brain cancer." He kept walking, his voice irritated. "I'm not incapacitated."

*Well, that's logical.* I rolled my eyes at his back, decided there was no point in arguing, and grabbed everything I could carry. I had to hustle to catch up with him.

At the exhibit area, Richard eyed our case and announced, "I need my drill. And the bits." I dashed back to the car, and as I hefted his big drill, I began to giggle, imagining how I would convince airport security that I wasn't a terrorist.


At his monthly chemo review with Dr. Klein, I confessed that Richard had lost ten pounds and that I considered that a personal failure. "Sometimes I have a hard time finding anything healthy to tempt his appetite," I said.

"Eating healthfully is important, just not when you're taking chemo." Dr. Klein smiled. "Ice cream, pudding, custard—anything that sounds good is fine, and the more calories, the better."

Richard grinned. "Is that a prescription?"

She laughed.


One balmy late-May morning, coffee cup in hand, Richard headed for his studio for the first time since before his radiation treatments. "I'm going to get out my rock-hauling cart and think," he said.

He had just started round four of chemo, and his spirits were high. I couldn't tell whether his buoyant mood was due to the antinausea medication or Dr. Klein's "prescription" to eat anything he wanted. It didn't matter. My spirits rose with his. *We can live with cancer*, I thought.

When I looked up from my writing, there sat my husband on one of the half dozen chiseled reddish sandstone blocks clustered near the kitchen garden, building stones salvaged from a demolished bank downtown where a young Richard had once licked fruit-flavored suckers while his father made deposits. Today's Richard sipped coffee, a smile on his tan face. A weathered canvas bucket hat shaded his shaved head and that sinuous surgery scar. A metal measuring tape was clipped to his belt; calipers, a mechanical pencil, and reading glasses protruded from his shirt pocket. The tripod crane he used for lifting smaller boulders stood ready.

Tears stung my eyes. Richard among his rocks, contemplating a new sculpture, would once have been normal. Now it looked like a miracle.

*Richard . . .*
*Saw birds everywhere.*
*Now, chisel in hand, sees art*
*Waiting in dark stone.*
—In a note from writer John Calderazzo

Over lunch, Richard reported that he had selected the sandstone block for the base of the mailbox sculpture he was planning. He pointed out the window at the largest block in the group, about three feet long, a foot and a half wide, and two-plus feet tall. "It's the most symmetrical, with the flattest top and bottom."

That afternoon, Richard fastened a sling around the block, raised the 450-pound stone with the chain hoist fastened under the apex of the tripod, and then lowered the block carefully onto the flatbed cart.

"It's poised for the next step," he said when he came inside. "And I'm ready for a nap."

The next morning, Richard rolled his gantry, a hand-powered horizontal crane he had invented for maneuvering unwieldy rocks, to the front yard. He attached the block to hoists suspended from the gantry's steel I beam and lifted the stone, turned it upside down in midair, and drilled four holes in the bottom. After epoxying a rebar "root" into each hole, he turned the block right side up again. Then he came inside to talk with me about placement.

"You're ready to dig the hole?" I was surprised.

Richard smiled. "Finally—if you recall, this was to be your birthday present."

"It's only May. My birthday isn't till September."

"It was for last year." His tone was dry, but he was smiling.

I hugged him, feeling positively giddy that he was sculpting again. "I forgot that. What I recall is that *you* were my birthday present—I got to spring you from the hospital."

While the concrete foundation for the mailbox sculpture cured, we drove to Denver for Richard's monthly appointment with Dr. Klein.


"You look great." Her smile was proud; the scale showed that he had regained those ten pounds.

"I haven't missed ice cream for breakfast since I last saw you."

"I hate you," she responded, not missing a beat.

We all cracked up. I turned away to swipe at tears. My love was back.

From Denver, we drove 835 miles to northwest Arkansas to visit Richard's family. When we reached his sister, Tish's, house, I felt her relief at seeing his vigorous walk and hearing his deep laugh. After dinner, he pulled out his juggling balls to entertain Oliver, Tish's young grandson. The next morning, Richard and his brother went out for a "boys' breakfast." Later, we visited his mother, who cried when she saw Richard.

"Son, you look so good! I was afraid you were dying!" She trembled as he hugged her.

I shook off a spurt of anger. He *was* dying. We all are—and also living.

Just before we crossed into mountain time on the way home, I spotted a crow-size, marbled-brown shorebird sporting a ridiculously long, down-curved bill.

"Long-billed curlew!"

Richard braked, whipped a U-turn, and drove back. Named for their rising, two-note *coo-LI* call, these shorebirds were once so common, they were shot by the score for restaurant fare. Icons of disappearing prairie wetlands, long-billed curlews are now so rare that we had seen them only twice before.

We watched as the curlew lifted into the air on pointed wings and flew low over the shortgrass prairie in a zigzagging pattern until it disappeared. "I hope it finds a mate," I said.

"We did."

Richard took my hand and turned the car west again, toward home.

*curlew*
*plumage streaked like prairie grasses*
*zigzags into summer*

# chapter twelve

## Day Thirteen

### Odometer Reading: 2,415 Miles

Sunday morning, Molly and Mark took us to brunch at a café on the bay to celebrate my fifty-fifth birthday. We sat outside, Richard in his brown pile hoodie, I wrapped in a gray wool sweater coat, reveling in the salty tang of sea air. Gulls cried as they foraged nearby; sea lions barked in the distance. Nearby, the clock on the tower of the Ferry Building chimed the hour, summoning a childhood memory.

I gripped the rail of the ferryboat as it neared the dock at the Ferry Building. The bay breeze ruffled my short hair. I was ten; Mom and Bill and I were on our way to the city to meet Granddad Milner for lunch. At Fisherman's Wharf, we scooped succulent crab with spicy sauce from paper cups, licking our fingers. Then we followed our noses uphill to the Ghirardelli Chocolate factory. Grandad gave Bill and me each a quarter. I selected a green foil tube containing chocolate dots in a mix of mint, milk, dark, and caramel and savored those morsels the whole ferry ride back across the bay.

Mom's health declined over the course of that spring of Richard's chemo, even as his improved. When we arrived at Mom and Dad's apartment one April morning to take them to the Brown Palace Hotel for high tea to celebrate Mom's seventy-eighth birthday, she was cranky.

"I can't find anything in this kitchen." She glared at me. "Nothing is where I expect it to be." Her tone implied it was my fault.

"I'm sorry," I said, puzzled because she had supervised us as we'd carefully transferred the contents of each cabinet and drawer to the identical place in the new apartment.

I helped Mom into her sweater. Her English-rose skin was gray, her limbs painfully thin. Something was seriously wrong. I needed to talk to Dad.

At the opulent Brown Palace, Mom settled with a sigh into the silk armchair Dad held out, and then my always decisive mother handed the elaborate menu to me. "You order."

She perked up when our server brought out a three-level stand loaded with warm scones, tiny sandwiches, and iced petits fours. "Happy birthday!" The server set a mini–sponge cake with a candle on it in front of Mom and pinned an orchid corsage to her turtleneck. "Thank you." Mom smiled, her blue eyes sparkling.

Mom had always loved sweets—I swear, she could smell a bakery from miles away. Now, after eating a few bites, she leaned back, eyes closed, fork idle. I touched her hand—it was freezing. She looked frighteningly fragile.

Back at their apartment, I pulled Dad aside.

"I'm really worried about Mom," I said bluntly. "Did you talk to Dr. Schorr?"

He looked guilty. "I forgot."

"When is her next appointment?"

"Next month." His eyes didn't quite meet mine.

*What isn't he telling me?* Dad didn't lie any more skillfully than I did. I vowed I'd follow up—later. Right then, I needed to get Richard home to rest up for his next round of chemo.

Caregivers constantly triage demands on our time and attention; we simply never have enough of either. The term "triage" came into use in the 1930s, when the U.S. Army began ranking the severity of soldiers' battlefield injuries. Those with the most critical needs were treated first; the rest waited. Caregiving often feels like battlefield medicine, and whether we are conscious of it or not, we rank every demand based on urgency. (Our own needs, of course, come last.) So, too, with caring for this planet and its living community. As philosopher and climate activist Kathleen Dean Moore said in a 2018 talk, "Even if it breaks our hearts, we have to confront again that existential question: What do we love too much to lose?" It's an impossible dilemma. No wonder guilt haunts us.

Just before Richard's fifth round of chemo, we hit the road again, this time for Carpenter Ranch in northwestern Colorado, where we had been granted a two-year "service residency," part uninterrupted time to pursue our own work, part service to reenvision a half acre of unused lawn as an interpretive landscape. We were excited about the opportunity to meld our heart work: my passion for plants and restorying the land, and Richard's innate understanding of design and sculpture. The residency also offered time out from cancer treatment.

It's easy to be consumed by a crisis, to let it engulf our lives the way a forest fire seems to swallow a landscape, the searing flames reducing to smoking ruins what was familiar. Only if we do, we miss the green sprouts of life poking through the ash and the renewal they promise. We miss finding hope, not blind optimism, hope that sees the "openings" in catastrophic change, "an embrace of the unknown and the unknowable," as Rebecca Solnit writes in *Hope in the Dark*.

Our proposal for the Carpenter Ranch garden envisioned a landscape design that would honor the history of the ranch and the surrounding river valley, ash and all. That story began with the Ute Indians, who named the river Yampa for the starchy root of a local wildflower and called the valley home until settlers pushed them out. We imagined structures evoking local geology and architecture—including the hulking, noisy presence of the nearby coal-fired power plant; gardens showcasing edible and heritage plants; and a native meadow that would breathe wildness into a cultivated landscape, reviving the community and stories inherent in the land.

There was precious little wildness in the suburbs north of Chicago where I grew up. The tallgrass prairie, that living tapestry of head-high grasses that novelist Willa Cather celebrated, had long been plowed, its rich soil turned to corn farms. By the time I was born, in 1956, the suburban grid was erasing those farm fields, too. Ironically, each yard boasted its own field-like monoculture of lawn tamed by droning mowers and poisonous chemicals. Trucks cruising through our neighborhood at dusk in summer sprayed a fog of DDT to nuke the hordes of insects—and, as Rachel Carson warned in *Silent Spring*, also killed the birds that fed on them.

My favorite spot was a shady little garden outside the kitchen door, where my mother planted rescued woodland wildflowers we dug up on surreptitious forays to vacant lots scheduled for development. Crimson wake-robin, snowy white trillium, blue forget-me-not, goldenrod . . . We nestled each plant carefully in our bike baskets as we pedaled them home.

The rest of my childhood yard was as tidy as our neighbors' yards, if less drenched in chemicals. A neatly edged lawn was bordered by flower beds that Mom filled with favorites from my grandparents' gardens: fragrant peonies in pink, ruby red, and white; drifts of lily of the valley, with their bell-shaped, sweet-scented blossoms; sunny yellow daffodils and purple grape hyacinths; tall hollyhocks whose flowers I transformed into frilly-skirted ballerinas. At the far end of the backyard, a tidy rectangle sprouted a vegetable garden inspired by the World War II victory gardens Mom and Dad grew up with. Rows of crunchy kohlrabi, parsnips, Swiss chard with bright red stalks, ruffled green-leaf lettuce, pink radishes . . . No one else I knew grew their own food. That embarrassed me as a child, but now I appreciate it.

That yard, with its sanctuary for wildflowers displaced by development, its edible plants, and its borders displaying heritage ornamentals, shaped my landscape aesthetic (except for the lawn). Every place where Richard, Molly, and I lived, I planted a patch of natives, added favorite perennials, and sowed a kitchen garden, even if only a tub of greens on a patio.

When we moved to Salida and bought our junky industrial property, I finally had a place to root and bloom (pun intended).

Before the backhoe dug the house foundation, I seeded swaths of native mountain prairie in what would be the front and side yards. During construction, I planted an edible garden just outside the kitchen-to-be in raised beds Richard built where above-ground oil tanks had once stood. Once the house was built, I filled borders in the front courtyard with neighborhood heritage plants: lilac bushes, peonies, oriental poppies, and daffodils. My mother loved that yard. I imagined a similar aesthetic for Carpenter Ranch, a garden that would honor both the wild community of the land and the people who inhabited it.

I called my parents as Richard drove us north to Carpenter on that late-June day.

"I miss being able to get away like that," said Mom. "Where is Carpenter Ranch?"

Dad reminded her that they had visited on a birding trip years before.

"I remember." Her voice turned testy. Then, to me, she said, "Maybe you can take us sometime."

*Oh, Mom!* "This isn't a vacation." I gentled my voice with an effort. "We're working."

"That's okay," she said airily. "We can entertain ourselves."

Once, they could have. For Dad's eightieth birthday two summers before, the family had gathered at a backcountry yurt. Mom and Dad hiked in with us, hand in hand. Mom picked out the constellations at night and delighted in the wildflowers and dawn bird chorus. That was then. Now, if we brought them to Carpenter, I knew there would be no time-out for me.

After the call, I stared out the car window. The highway

wound downhill through shadowed forests and sunlit meadows, following the cascading Eagle River. The tires hummed.

"You're quiet," Richard said.

I sighed. "Mom wants us to bring them to Carpenter Ranch."

"No way!" He spoke so firmly that I laughed.

"Thanks. She's so needy now. I don't think she grasps what we're going through."

He reached for my hand. "You're right: She doesn't understand what you're going through. I wish I didn't need you to tend to me. But thank you for doing it."

I leaned over and kissed him. "I love you. I feel lucky to have you in my life."

We settled into the Bunkhouse, a one-room cabin next to the historic ranch house and interpretive center. The resonant calls of sandhill cranes woke us at dawn. In the midday heat, clouds of swallows chattered through the air, scooping up mouthfuls of mosquitoes; after sunset, mouse-eared bats squeaked and flickered in pursuit of the same prey. We interviewed Betsy and Geoff, the ranch managers, and read accounts of ranch life and valley history; we explored the buildings and wandered a trail along the looping Yampa River. We were connecting to the place; a design would emerge as we learned its stories.

After dinner on our final evening there, I opened *Still Alice,* a novel from my book stack. I read into the night, absorbed in the tale of a professor descending into Alzheimer's disease. I woke in the morning with tears on my cheeks.

"What's wrong?" Richard woke and pulled me into his arms.

"It's Mom." I gulped. "The character in the book. Her confusion and anxiety, the shift in her personality from cheery to irritable, her emotional distance."

"Oh." He stroked my back, evaluating. "I can see that. I can definitely see that."

I wiped my eyes and blew my nose. "What will we do?"

"Get her tested. Then do our best. It's all we can do."

He kissed me and rubbed my shoulders. Then another kiss, longer and deeper. I let myself drift into lovemaking, lost in the moment. It just wasn't long enough.

Back home, Richard began his next cycle of chemo and we prepared for Cabefest, our annual party to celebrate the July birthdays of Richard, his older brother, Ron, and my dad. This year, we were celebrating Richard's sixtieth and what we thought was his recovery from brain cancer. Molly flew in from San Francisco with Mark. Bill and Lucy drove in from Washington state, bringing high school–age Alice; Connor, their eldest grandson; and Mom and Dad from Denver. Richard's sister arrived from Arkansas with her friend Juana; Cabe nephews and nieces and their families gathered as well. The influx filled our house and cottage, two borrowed Airstream trailers parked by Richard's studio, and Ron and Bonnie's house across town.

On Cabefest morning, a crowd gathered for a champagne brunch and a boule tournament. *Boule* ("ball" in French) is similar to bocce, only played on gravel and using steel balls, which inspire all manner of ribald jokes. Richard beamed as he greeted everyone and recruited teams for his favorite game. I stayed busy replenishing food and drinks and tending Mom, who had once enjoyed our parties and now was anxious and unsettled.

Later, everyone gathered in the shade of the living room porch to sing "Happy Birthday." A raven perched on the roof, as if listening. Richard, stretched full-length on the chaise, grinned. "I'm a lucky guy."

After breakfast the next morning, Richard and Molly talked on the porch, Dad and Bill went birding, and everyone else packed. Mom settled herself onto a stool at the kitchen counter as I finished cleaning up from the meal.

"I'm hungry," she announced.

I stared at her, open-mouthed. She had just eaten.

"I'm hungry," she repeated, like a baby bird, beak agape.

I considered. "Would you like a sandwich? I need to make lunches for the drive."

"Where are we going?"

"Home."

"Are you coming, too? I don't want to go if you're not coming."

*Fuck.* "I can't, Mom." I chose my words carefully, torn between exhaustion and tears. "I have to stay here and take care of Richard."

"But you'll come visit soon, won't you?"

"We will, Mom. We always do."

"That's right. You always do."

Later, I repeated our conversation to Bill and Lucy. "You've got to talk to Dad," I said. "He isn't listening to me."

Bill looked sad. "You're right. I'll talk to him."

Lucy hugged me. "I'm sorry."

"Me too." I was overwhelmed: Mom with Alzheimer's, cared for by Dad, who was legally blind, depending on me and Richard, still recovering from brain cancer. It was too much.

A week later, Richard looked up from his postbreakfast coffee. "I've got the garden-arbor commission figured out." He sketched an elegant upright arc of curving wire fence panel held in tension between four square wood posts, each topped with a rounded river-rock "finial" held up by ordinary galvanized plumbing pipe.

I smiled. "It's a modern, terraphiliac twist on arts-and-crafts design. They'll love it."

"I think it'll only take a few days." He grinned. "Of course, that's what I always say."

The next morning, Richard packed his tools and materials and drove to the client's house to begin installation, leaving me a whole glorious day to just write. That evening over his Belgian-style ale and my sparkling water with lime, he regaled me with stories and then threw back his head and laughed. "Thank you."

"For what?"

"For nudging me back to work. It feels good. I'm tired, but I feel stronger than I have in a long time. And thank you for making my meals, tending the household, and growing our food."

He sounded so like the Richard of old—fully engaged in life —I had to blink away tears.


That Friday, July 16, was Richard's sixtieth birthday. He spent the day at the Colorado Metalsmithing Association's annual conference, which featured a talk by sculptor-blacksmith Albert Paley, one of Richard's art heroes. He was jazzed when he got home. "I'm going to finish celebrating my birthday with a swim in the river."

"Are you sure you're up for that?" An avid swimmer, he hadn't been in the water since before the birds, and he had never swum in the swift and snowmelt-cold Arkansas River.

"I'm sure," he said. I debated about trying to discourage him, but once he made up his mind . . . I grabbed my camera, and we walked the three blocks to the river together.

Kayaks bobbed in the whitewater park; a bus full of preteens jammed the river walk, giggling and daring each other to dip their toes into the bracing water. They ignored the old guy with the shaved head and surgery scar until he dove straight in, provoking gasps of "Dude!"

Richard surfaced midchannel. I let out my breath. He shook the water out of his eyes like a dog, swam downstream, and then stroked smoothly back cross-current toward the riverbank where I stood. He climbed out to a round of applause and grinned at me.

"That felt great. I'm going to do it again." And he did.

In my favorite photo from that swim, Richard floats downstream on his back, smile broad, muscled arms sculling, as relaxed in the swift water as if he were seated in a porch rocker.

On the walk home, I took his hand. "Happy sixtieth—may you have many more."

"I feel good," he said, "as if that's a possibility again."

*river slaps tan skin*
*muscles bunch, stroking cross-current*
*your smile gleams*

# chapter thirteen

## Day Thirteen

### Odometer Reading: 2,533 Miles

After that birthday brunch in San Francisco, we headed south to meet a friend outside the Palo Alto Art Center. Richard and Louella sat in the shade and talked while I wandered through Patrick Dougherty's life-size "village" of conical cottages woven of willow branches, inhaling their earthy fragrance. When I looked over, Richard was gesturing with his hands, face animated; Louella listened with a smile so sad, it hurt my heart. She knew it was their last conversation.

Back on the highway, Richard slept until we wound uphill into the Santa Cruz Mountains, where coast redwoods towered overhead. He powered down his window. "I love the smell."

The sticky breeze whipped hair into my eyes, and I turned to ask him to close the window. He was smiling, eyes closed, breathing in redwoods—alive and savoring the moment. I shut my mouth.

Two weeks after Richard's sixtieth birthday and that river swim, we returned to Denver for his quarterly brain MRIs. When she greeted us the next morning, Dr. Klein didn't smile. I assumed she was still cranky about her own sixtieth birthday, just a few days after Richard's. They teased each other, he calling her "just a young thing," and she retorting that he would always be older.

It wasn't her birthday. Dr. Klein turned her computer monitor so we could view the MRI images and pointed to a circular white shadow in Richard's right temporal lobe: "It looks like a new tumor."

My heart stuttered.

"This is not the news any of us wanted," she said, her gaze steady. "I want a biopsy as soon as possible. What are your plans for the day?"

"Eat breakfast, visit my parents, and then head for home." I was firmly in denial.

"But we'll do whatever is needed," Richard added, as he took my hand.

"Go eat breakfast," Dr. Klein said. "I'll have Neurosurgery call you. In the meantime, what do you need?"

I needed a dose of vitamin N, nature. I looked at Richard. "Let's take a walk on the Sixth Avenue parkway." He nodded.

Dr. Klein's eyes glistened. "Call if you need me." She hugged Richard and then me.

"We'll be okay," I said quietly in her ear as he headed out the door.

"Me too," she responded. "But crap!"

"Yeah—crap."


Richard never craved wilderness time the way I do. We managed just one family backpacking trip, a weekend outing to the Dolly

Sods Wilderness Area, for my birthday that fall in West Virginia. Richard and four-year-old Molly were so miserable that I took pity on them after the first night, and we packed out. On the way home, we stopped for "real food," in Molly's words, and Richard's favorite dark-roast coffee. I never tried backpacking with them again.

Later that fall, Molly came down with mononucleosis. Tending her through weeks of feverish nights left Richard and me with no energy to tend our new marriage. By the time Molly returned to Colorado and her mother at Christmas, we were exhausted and distant—until Richard discovered a patch of undisturbed woods not far from our apartment and invited me to see it. We walked there as spring wildflowers exploded into bloom: yellow trout lily, purple dogtooth violet, and red wake-robin and white trillium that reminded me of my mother's wildflower garden. Perched side by side on a sandstone ledge amid the new green of oak, maple, and tulip trees leafing out, we sipped coffee from my old steel fieldwork thermos and talked, holding hands. There, in the woods, we healed.

There was no body of research then to explain what I knew instinctively: When things fall apart, get outside in the wild and soak up vitamin N, nature's medicine. It doesn't just boost our physical health. Time in nature is restorative for our brains, too, helping us learn and focus more easily and solve problems more creatively. We make better decisions and are less violent. Just viewing images of nature increases activity in the brain areas associated with empathy and altruism; simply walking outdoors in a natural setting reduces negative feelings and eases depression. Nature gives us back our best selves.

After Dr. Brega confirmed that the shadow in Richard's MRI was likely a new tumor, we sped across South Park on the road home, Richard at the wheel. I spotted a small group of pronghorn in the mountain prairie: "One buck, two does, two more does," and then "three fawns!"

Richard pulled off in a cloud of dust. The fawns stood half-hidden behind the does on long, spindly legs, heads turned toward us, black eyes huge, alert.

"Wow!" Richard grinned when I passed him the binoculars. "I've never seen a pronghorn fawn before."

I grinned back. "And here are three—like a gift."

That Sunday of our belated honeymoon trip, Richard fell asleep again as soon as we hit traffic in Santa Cruz. He woke when I stopped at a tidal inlet near Moss Landing. A snowy egret, all brilliant white atop skinny black legs, stood at the edge of the mudflat. I handed Richard the binoculars, and he smiled when his eyes found the bird. Beyond the egret, he spotted a sea otter floating on its back in open water. His smile grew. "Too bad we didn't bring the kayak," he said. "This would be a great place to paddle."

"It would." *If you could still paddle*, I thought, and swallowed the words.

The surgery to remove Richard's second brain tumor was scheduled for the week in mid-August when we had planned our second stay at Carpenter Ranch. I thought we should postpone; Richard suggested visiting Carpenter beforehand.

"Some peace and quiet will help me—you, too—prepare for

what's ahead. I'll bring my surveyor's tape and draw a site plan," he continued. "We'll collect stories. That'll give us something to work on while I recuperate. By next spring, we'll have a concept."

My eyes filled with tears. Richard patted his lap. I snuggled in.

"Hearing you say 'next spring' makes me sad and happy at the same time. This surgery scares me. I hope by next spring you're past brain cancer and we're walking on."

His arms tightened around me. "The surgery scares me, too, my love. But this is what we have. We'll walk the journey together."

Scared or not, I focused on making sure Richard was prepared for the surgery, mentally, emotionally, and physically—including preparing a profusion of anticancer food. When we set out for Carpenter Ranch the next week, the backseat of our Subaru looked like a farmers' market. There were crusty loaves of Richard's fragrant whole-wheat boule, individually packed servings of my homemade hot breakfast cereal, his favorite green tea, orange-infused dark chocolate, and other staples. One cooler overflowed with produce from our garden: lettuce, cucumbers, tomatoes, strawberries, and broccoli. The other held local cheese and peaches, homemade yogurt, green chiles, eggs from a neighbor's chickens, and bottles of Richard's favorite Belgian-style ale.

At the ranch, we met with a local garden club to gather plant lists and lore. The granddaughter of one of the ranch founders regaled us with stories, including the time the cowboys brought home a pair of orphaned bighorn-sheep kids. These rambunctious youngsters were given free rein in the ranch yard until they broke into the kitchen garden and ate everything—"even the rhubarb"—after which those two bighorn kids became dinner, already stuffed.

Walking back to the bunkhouse one afternoon, we watched a

rainbow appear, the bands of color growing brighter and more intense. When the shower reached us, we dashed to the cabin hand in hand, soaked and laughing. By the time we left for home, we had sketched out the new edible garden, and hope, Emily Dickinson's "thing with feathers," sang in my soul.

Then I called my parents. Mom, I learned, had fallen and broken her left arm.

"It's a hairline fracture too close to the shoulder joint for a cast," Dad reported. Mom had been sent to a rehabilitation center; Dad planned to visit during the day. "Joan is disoriented."

*Hell. What happened to my bright mother?*

"I love you," I said. "Thanks for taking care of Mom."

"Thanks for all your help."

I woke in the dark that night, heart racing, and curled around Richard's warm and comforting back. In two days, we would drive to Denver for his second brain surgery. And figure out what was going on with Mom. It was overwhelming. Then I remembered: Molly was flying in for the weekend. She would help. Relieved, I fell asleep again, remembering a few months before, when we were driving Mom and Dad to a doctor's appointment and I suggested that we hire someone to help them with meals and cleaning. To my great surprise, Mom, who had always resisted having help, agreed. Dad did not. "We're managing just fine," he said emphatically.

I sighed, unwilling to argue.

Then Molly spoke up. "I hope you'll take this as coming from someone who loves and cares about you." She put her arm around Dad, sitting next to her in the backseat of the car, and leaned forward to touch Mom's shoulder. "It seems to me that even if you don't think you need that kind of help, you could accept it as a gift from us, who love you. We can't be with you every day, and knowing you have help would keep us from worrying so much."

Mom nodded.

Dad said he would think about it.

*What a wise and loving person we raised*, I thought, brushing away tears.

In the morning, I called the rehab center. Mom asked about our trip. Then her voice turned childlike. "I don't know where I am. Can you come get me?"

I said gently, "You're at the rehab center for a few days. Remember?"

"I don't think Berto knows where I am." Her voice shook.

"Dad's on his way," I said.

"I think he called. I couldn't understand what he said."

Just then, I heard Dad walk in. Mom set the phone receiver down with a *thunk*.

"Dad!" I shouted into the phone. "Dad!" I heard fumbling noises and then his voice. I reported Mom's confusion. He promised to call her doctor. I tried not to worry.

The next afternoon, walking home in a mellow mood after a massage, I checked my messages and heard my mother's voice, as smug and defiant as any six-year-old's: "I'm home. So there!"

I looked up. Richard strode toward me. I walked straight into his arms.

"What's wrong?"

"My mother's home already."

"Oh." He leaned down and kissed me. "That's not good." He took my hand.

Later, I called Dad. "Joan's much more lucid now that she's home. We're fine. Don't worry."

I swallowed a snort. Mom had a broken arm and was confused; Dad, her primary caregiver, was legally blind. Figuratively, too, it seemed.

Our best work is fueled by active hope, when we embrace the unknown yet aim for a positive outcome, a positive impact on our lives and the life of this planet. Optimism helps, as do patience and tenacity. Hope is not believing blindly, as Dad clearly did. It means acting out of faith in the power of human creativity and community. Together, we can in fact work wonders.

"I wish I could drive. You could rest." Richard climbed into the passenger seat of the car. It was September, a month after his second brain surgery and the day before my fifty-fourth birthday. We were headed to Santa Fe for a weekend, our stay a birthday gift from our neighbors Kerry and Dave. The thirty-one stainless-steel staples that secured the Zipper, Richard's surgery scar, had been removed. But his vision was still doubled; the images from his two eyes didn't merge. He couldn't drive, read, or use his computer. The neuro-ophthalmologist had assured us that once the swelling from the surgery subsided—in a month or more—his vision would return to normal.

More worrisome to me was Richard's impaired sense of direction, a function of losing most of his right temporal lobe in the surgery. Walking home from the post office the day before, he had gotten lost on a route we had taken daily for years. He laughed as I aimed him in the right direction. I shivered, realizing I could no longer let him go anywhere by himself.

I blinked away tears. "You will be able to drive again, sweetie." *I hope.*

After settling into our corner room with a view over downtown Santa Fe's tile roofs, we walked through crisp evening air to a favorite café. Richard ordered a Santa Fe pale ale; I chose a glass of champagne. "Happy birthday!" Richard said, as we clinked glasses. Then his smile dimmed. "I'm sorry we're not at Aspen Ridge." We had canceled the residency—again.

"This weekend counts as time out, my sweetie," I lied, without even a twinge of conscience. And then added truthfully, "I'm grateful to be here with you."

Those three days were heaven. We lounged in the shade of the hotel's veranda to read, write, and sketch. We walked to galleries and art museums; we explored parks and hung out at coffeehouses; we devoured chile-infused meals. We slept late and made leisurely love, the windows open to ravens croaking and the deep voices of the bells from the nearby cathedral. It felt like we were coming alive again.

Our last night in Santa Fe, I called my folks. Dad answered and then handed the phone to Mom. "I can't hold it," she said. I heard Dad's voice, muffled: "Can you hear her now?"

*Shit.* Mom had forgotten how to use a phone.

"We're in Santa Fe, Mom, right downtown," I said, my voice too cheerful. "I can hear the cathedral bells."

"How nice. Are you giving a talk there?"

"We're here to celebrate my birthday."

"You had a birthday—how nice." Her tone was as flat as if she were commenting on the weather. "I'm tired. Goodbye!"

I held the phone to my ear, listening to nothing. My mother, the one who always sent a birthday card with a note written in her crabbed hand, who always called, who more than once had embarrassed me by singing "Happy Birthday" in public—that mother was gone. I knew intellectually what Alzheimer's meant, but still, I was not prepared for this profound loss.

Richard looked up from his book. "What's wrong?"

I walked over, sat on his lap, and buried my face in his shoulder. He put his arms around me.

"She's gone," I said, and tears slid down my face.

He nodded, his cheek against my hair. "There's a large sense in which the mother you knew, your champion, the one who loved the particulars of you, is gone. I'm sorry."

I lifted my damp face for a kiss. We sat watching the sunset as ravens flapped past. The bells of the cathedral rang the hour. We walked downstairs, hand in hand, and out into the mild night as the first stars pricked the dark sky.

*ravens croak autumn*
*cathedral bells ring*
*time ... time ... time*

# chapter fourteen

### Day Fourteen

Odometer Reading: 2,654 Miles

That Monday of the Big Trip we didn't hit the road until noon, but there was no rush: Lucia Lodge, our night's destination, lay only fifty-seven winding miles down Highway 1. As I drove, Richard munched calamari left from the previous night's dinner, a napkin protecting his favorite cranberry Pendleton shirt from spills. Our first stop was in Carmel, where we visited the mission my artist great-grandmother sketched in 1924, when the surrounding land still sprouted tidy fields and blooming orchards.

Next was a pullout where steep cliffs plunged into a cove we called Otter Cove to commemorate the first time we had seen sea otters together, years before. Richard was so eager to spot otters that he opened the door before the car had stopped. I braked, grabbed his leftovers and napkin, and handed him the binoculars. He hauled himself upright and leaned against the hood to scan the fog-gray water below, laced with ivory foam from dashing against the cliffs.

I shrugged on a fleece jacket and climbed out as Richard said, "There!"

He pointed toward several dark shapes in a patch of kelp about fifty yards off the rocks. "Are those otter heads?"

One turned and rolled smoothly into a dive, answering his question. "Good spot!" I said.

A grin transformed Richard's swollen face as he watched the two remaining otters bob in the swells, front paws tucked across their chests. Then he handed me the binoculars and folded himself back into the car. I buckled his seat belt, tucked his napkin back into the neck of his shirt, and handed him his lunch. "Onward," he said. "I'll watch for condors."

On a sunny March day three springs later, Molly, our friend Laura, and I scanned the parking lot at Otter Cove to make sure no one was looking, and then I clambered over the head-high chain-link fence. On the other side, I scattered a bagful of Richard's ashes over the cliffs, returning a bit of him—now pale grit on the breeze—to consort with the sea otters he loved.

Driving home from Santa Fe, we turned aside at Bandelier National Monument and ate lunch in the shade of box elder trees along Frijoles Creek. A foraging red-breasted nuthatch serenaded us with its *Yank! Yank! Yank!* calls. After our picnic, we rambled along a quiet trail and stopped to sniff the platelike bark of a ponderosa pine tree so fat that Richard's long arms stretched barely halfway around its trunk. Its distinctive vanilla fragrance perfumed still, hot air.

"Why does the tree spend the energy to produce the fragrance?" Richard asked, as we walked hand in hand back to the car.

"I'm not sure anyone knows," I said, "but I'd guess the aromatic compounds are defenses of some sort. That huge trunk offers a sizable food resource for any critter who can figure out how to digest the lignin and cellulose."

"I love the smell." He swung our linked hands high. "It always makes me smile."

"Seeing your smile is a gift."

"Am I still moody?"

"Some," I said carefully.

Richard didn't prefer to notice his "blue" moods. I couldn't tell whether the dark times resulted from the altered geography of his brain and his missing right temporal lobe, or from learning he had terminal brain cancer, or from both.

"It doesn't feel like that to me." His voice was defensive.

"I know, sweetie." I squeezed his hand. "It's harder for you to be aware now."

As we drove north along the muddy Rio Grande, Richard said, "Brooke said they wouldn't remove anything that would affect my personality."

I marshaled patience before replying. "Remember what Dr. Brega said about the brain not being like a map with fixed boundaries between the sections? And how each brain is different?"

He was quiet for so long, I thought he had gone to sleep. Warm sun poured through the windshield. Cottonwood trees showed hints of autumn amber. Directly ahead of us, a solitary cumulus cloud billowed in the brilliant blue sky. Suddenly it threw out a lightning bolt, followed by a crack of thunder, as electrical energy superheated the air.

"Maybe we should read that brain book Nancy and Dave sent." Richard's voice startled me almost as much as the thunder. "It might help us both understand."

I gripped the steering wheel as a gust shook the car. "I'm sorry I'm not more patient."

"I don't want to be a source of frustration. I want to be a source of support and joy."

Tears blurred the road ahead. "You are in many ways, my sweetie," I said. He was also often frustrating, but I didn't say that. It wasn't his fault his brain was impaired.

The cloud released another bolt of lightning. Rain splattered down, turned to pounding hail, and then turned back to rain so hard the wipers couldn't keep up. Then the rain quit as suddenly as it had begun and we emerged into dazzling sunshine.

"That's how life feels to me right now," Richard said.

"Unpredictable? Buffeting you around?"

"Pretty much."

"Oh, my sweetie! I'm sorry. What should we do?"

"I've been thinking about going on a weeklong meditation retreat, if you think that's a good idea."

"Absolutely."

A meditation retreat would help Richard's brain continue to heal. Brain research shows that meditation acts like doses of nature, boosting our ability to focus, learn, and make healthy decisions, and strengthening our empathy circuits. We can all use that.

At home, I unpacked the car and then went to work in the yard—my form of meditation—while Richard took a nap. As an introvert living in a body studded with what feel like hundreds of tiny antennae tuned to nonverbal signals, I am easily overwhelmed by the stimuli of my fellow humans: our voices and words, the noise of our devices, our volatile emotions, and the electricity of our metabolic energy. Vitamin N time, specifically the company of plants, settles me. These green beings actively sense and respond to the world around them, and communicate using an aromatic vocabulary of dispersed organic chemicals. What soothes me is knowing that these "breathing buddies," as the poet Clifford Burke writes, are Earth's life-support system and perhaps our most important defense against global climate change. Plants exhale as waste the oxygen we must inhale, and inhale the carbon dioxide that we and our industrial processes off-gas. Our interdependence is evident in every breath we take.

Plants also grow our planet's living infrastructure, providing food and shelter for all. I admire their self-sufficiency, the way they use the simplest and most common materials—carbon dioxide, water and minerals, and the sun's energy—to make their own food, the complex sugars that also feed every other life on Earth, directly or indirectly.

What makes vitamin N, plants and all, so effective in reweaving selves unraveled by the fevered pace and crises of our times is that nature models resilience. The interdependent community of species that animates this blue planet is biased to continue living, no matter what humans are screwing up. In the midst of our mess, the big sagebrush dotting the grasslands around our house keeps inhaling carbon dioxide and respiring oxygen, the mountain bluebirds still hunt grasshoppers, the potted amaryllis on the windowsill continues to bloom. Knowing that life as a whole goes on about its business—perhaps not unchanged but not defeated, either—is a heartening reminder that the world turns on something more substantive and lasting than human travails: the spark of existence that animates this third rock from the sun.

Nature in the form of the restored prairie in our yard provided the balm I needed to survive the wild journey with Richard's brain cancer.

"I'm not going to commit suicide," Richard said, and took a sip of his Belgian ale.

It was November, almost two months after that birthday trip to Santa Fe. Late sun poured golden light over peaks visible out our living-room windows. Flames crackled in the woodstove.

I stared at the man I had lived with and loved for twenty-eight years, my mouth agape at his words.

He calmly scooped a tortilla chip into the guacamole I had just made and popped chip and dip into his mouth. He chewed deliberately and then added, "We talked about it. Remember? I've decided not to. I don't want to leave a gory body for you to clean up."

I did remember. And I had to clamp down on anger again. Richard had brought up suicide after Doctor Klein told us the tumors had returned. "Maybe I'll just kill myself before things get bad," he said that morning, as we walked hand in hand through the crowded halls of the hospital. "That way, you wouldn't have to take care of me."

I grabbed Richard's arm and looked up, pinning his gaze. "Don't even think that! It's ugly. I'm with you to the end, whatever and whenever that is."

"It seems logical to me." He was genuinely puzzled, Mars— the intellectual whose right brain was impaired—trying to understand the now-foreign language of Venus's emotions.

I took a deep breath and did my best to calm down. Richard seemed to view suicide clinically, as a tool to spare us from having to live with his dying.

"I get that, but it's not, sweetie," I said. "Trust me. Suicide is a bad idea, for you and for me, and for Molly. It leaves a trail of pain."

He frowned. "I'll think about that."

"You do that. And talk to me. I don't want to be surprised."

At home, I repeated the conversation to our friends Kerry and Dave. Dave was quiet. Kerry, a former lawyer, was stunned, then angry. "Why would he even think that? It's crazy! And cruel!"

"I think it seemed tidy," I said, suddenly weary. "As if he could time his death and save me the trouble of dealing with it."

She shook her head. "It's a crazy idea! Does he know that?"

I sighed. "It makes sense to a guy living only in the logical side of his brain. The side that understands emotions is pretty seriously impaired. He's trying to take care of me."

"Do you want Dave to talk to him?"

Dave looked at Kerry with horror, as if to say, *Thanks a lot!*

I chuckled and felt my tension ease. "I don't think so. But thanks."

Now, I sipped my sparkling water while I thought about Richard's pronouncement. Apparently, he had been considering suicide all along without mentioning it.

His not talking about suicide probably resulted from his lost temporal lobe and lost awareness. Also from being a strong guy whose instinct was to protect me, whether I preferred it or not. I didn't always consult him, either—out of hyperawareness, wanting to shield him from the worst. Different motivations, same effect: a partnership based on what Richard the economist called "asymmetric information." Knowledge not shared by both sides is no longer equal.

"I'm glad you've decided against it." I tried to read his face, to ascertain whether he really had given up the idea. I couldn't tell. I made a mental note to ask again after a few weeks, to check in more often and do my best to listen with an open mind.

Richard's very male habit of retreating to uncommunicative silence had always frustrated me, as I'm sure my very female habit of expressing my feelings out loud—sometimes very out loud—frustrated him. He prized maintaining a calm exterior, no matter what he was feeling inside. He turned inward to process his thoughts and emotions; I tended to leap based on intuitions I couldn't always articulate clearly. The challenges of our first married year exacerbated those differences: two cross-country moves in nine months, first from Wyoming to West Virginia, and then to Washington state; Molly's illness, followed by her return to her mother in Colorado; Richard's resignation from his academic post with no other job in sight. By the end of that summer, when we moved in with Bill and family, I was frazzled and Richard had withdrawn.

I didn't mind his need to think things through; I minded that he made decisions for the two of us without consulting me. On a walk one night, Richard let slip that his suggestion to move to Washington resulted from his fear that our marriage was failing. He had decided that I needed to live near my brother because, he said calmly, "you'd have family to take care of you."

I was stunned. "It didn't occur to you to ask me how I felt or where I wanted to live?"

"No," he said, all reason. "I figured if we split up, Bill would be there for you."

I took a deep breath. Then another. I was still mad. "While

you and Molly head for her mother's house in Colorado, I'm going backpacking at home in Wyoming. I need to think."

Richard accused me of running away. I held my ground. "We can talk afterward," I said, unsure of what "afterward" would bring but sure of my need for time alone in the wilderness, where I would be able to hear my inner voice without interference. I knew I loved Richard and Molly; I didn't know if our fledgling blended family could survive our differences.

And now here he was, a once sensitive guy whose remodeled brain seemed to have forgotten to communicate. Adjusting to a physical decline is especially difficult for men used to depending on their strength, men raised in families or cultures where talking about emotions is a weakness. Honestly, it's hard for any of us. We don't take gracefully to losing capabilities that have defined our sense of who we are.

We don't take gracefully to change, period. Living with our hearts outstretched in difficult times engages our compassion and empathy circuits and calms our fight-or-flight responses, helping us to be less reactive and more creative and thoughtful. More likely to see the nuances of any situation and a wider range of choices, and to craft a positive outcome.

The afternoon after Richard's bombshell about deciding not to commit suicide, we headed to Denver for his monthly appointments. He took the wheel. Snowflakes streamed across the road in feathery lines. I spotted a herd of pronghorn, ivory butts turned to the wind. "I hope they winter well."

"I hope they move downhill before winter," Richard responded. "Their genes have been shaped by several millennia of experience with these winters. I expect they know what they're doing."

"I wish I could say the same," he said.

"About knowing what you're doing?" He nodded. I reached over. "I'm sorry, my sweetie. I wish I could wave my magic wand and make you well. Does it help to be walking this journey together?"

"It does. Save your magic wand. Just give me your love, even when it's hard. I need that."

"I'm doing my best. I'm not perfect, as you know. But I always love you."

He smiled. It felt like the sun emerging after months of gray. "Thank you. It helps."

At the VA hospital the next morning, Dr. Klein tapped Richard's knees to check his synapses and tested his grip, wincing a little at the strength in his fingers.

Then she smiled. "I have good news: Your most recent MRI shows no sign of tumor recurrence." She added, "The longer you stay tumor-free, the lower your chances of recurrence."

Richard reached for my hand. We grinned at each other.

"We used to think of diabetes as a death sentence," she said. "But now we know it's something people can live with, and live well. Think of your brain cancer that way: Keep up your wellness routine and do what feels good to you. Live, brain cancer and all."

"How's your juggling?" she asked.

At the previous appointment, when Dr. Klein had asked how Richard was feeling, he had reached into his briefcase, pulled out three colored balls, tossed them into the air, and begun to juggle. After a moment, he'd lifted one foot, juggling balls still circling.

Dr. Klein laughed. "Can I show you off?"

He nodded, caught the balls, followed her into the hall, and resumed juggling.

"Braun! Look at this!" A man's head poked out the doorway across the hall. He grinned and came out, bringing another doc with him. Soon a crowd of oncology staff collected, smiles blooming.

"Any day you can make your oncologist laugh is a really good day," Richard said later.

That November day, Richard said, "I didn't bring my juggling balls this time."

"Next time, I want to see you juggle overhand," Dr. Klein said.

"I'll do that," he responded, smile growing.

"Now get out of here and do something fun. I don't need to see you until January." Dr. Klein's smile included me. We hugged her, wished her happy holidays, and headed out of the building hand in hand, stunned in a good way this time.

"I have to pee," Richard announced. We were only a few miles past Otter Cove. I spotted a state-park sign ahead, turned into the dusty parking lot, and helped Richard out of the car.

He reached for his fly and then said, "Rule number two: No peeing in public."

"Right," I said, suddenly teary. "The toilets are just beyond that fence."

There was no gate, just a stile. Once, Richard would have bounded up the wooden steps without a second thought. Now, I went first, backward, and held both of his hands, steadying his wobbling progress.

On the way back, Richard stopped at the top of the stile. He let go of my hands and stretched his arms overhead, grinning. I held my breath, bracing to catch him. He was steady in his joy, for the moment.

*Highway 1*
*fog to sunshine to fog again*
*ocean breathes in time*

# chapter fifteen

*Day Fifteen*

## Odometer Reading: 2,681 Miles

We stopped for a picnic lunch at a familiar trailhead in Andrew Molera State Park. On past trips, we had rambled along a sandy track through spreading oak trees, past a stand of fragrant eucalyptus where ranch buildings had once stood, and out to a beach. Now, sitting at a picnic table in the shade of an octopus-armed oak tree, Richard chuckled. I looked up from preparing our simple meal of crusty bread and gouda cheese, with coleslaw and a sliced pear. "What's funny?"

"Remember that time with Dida when the California towhee lured her into the poison oak? And then we washed her under the pump? And she shook and soaked us both?"

Dida (short for Perdida, "Lost One" in Spanish) was the stray shar-pei with the ebullient personality who had followed us home one night when we lived in New Mexico. She had picked us, her wagging tail and wriggling body seemed to say, and that was that. On the day Richard recalled, a towhee, a brown bird that looks like a large, drab sparrow, was chip-chip-trilling from the dense growth of poison oak along the trail. Dida, fascinated by the sound, burrowed into the thicket, coating her fur with the plants' skin-irritating oil, and then, when we tried to rinse her off, soaked us as she shook her loose skin, flinging water and poison-oak oil everywhere.

The first time we made love that Wyoming winter when we met, Richard pulled me close afterward, tears in his eyes. "Thank you," he said. "I know what love feels like now." My heart melted. Here was my perfect guy: brilliant and also tender, vulnerable and kind —everything I dreamed of. I hadn't yet met the Richard who could aim angry words as precisely and deliberately as a scalpel blade, and who would stew about a fight for weeks.

Growing up the dreamy and artistic middle son in a family proud of its white-collar status, Richard baffled his relatives. After he finished his PhD, his mother often reminded him that he had failed high school algebra—twice. Neither of his parents made it past high school—not uncommon for the times, but I suspect Mr. Raymond would have excelled if he had gotten the opportunity. Mr. Raymond's father, a Methodist preacher, died of tuberculosis when my father-in-law was an infant. The seven kids all helped support the family. I once asked him if he remembered his first job.

"Shining shoes for the neighbors," he said, without a pause.

"How old were you?" I asked.

"About four, I reckon."

Mr. Raymond "drove truck" after high school, trained pilots during World War II, and worked in supply-chain management in mining, a career that took him and Miss Alice and the growing family from Arkansas to Salida when Richard was one. When his middle son preferred hunting rocks and daydreaming to excelling in school, Mr. Raymond's experience with poverty made him a harsh father—I think he worried that Richard would fail in life, too. Hence the confrontation on the church porch that long-ago night in Texas. The rift that opened still hadn't mended when I met Richard.

Coming from a close-knit family, I grieved Richard's estrangement from his father and looked for ways to bridge it. Then, in the spring of 2004, we learned that Mr. Raymond had been diagnosed with terminal lung disease. "You need to go," I said.

Richard's jaw tightened. "I'm busy. Flights to Arkansas are expensive."

"I know that." We were settled in Salida; Richard's consulting work was booming. "But he's your father. This could be your last chance."

Richard turned away without speaking.

A week later, he flew to Arkansas, where his dad decided to enter hospice care at home. Each month after that, we drove the 1,200 miles to the folks' house with Isis, our Great Dane, to help for a week. Richard and his dad gradually began to talk, finding common ground in their mutual love for Salida.

"Do you bank at First State?" Mr. Raymond asked one morning, after lowering himself onto the couch in the family room. He twitched the hose of his oxygen tank into a precise S curve at his feet. Isis raised her huge head. I set down my knitting and stroked her silky black ears.

Richard looked up from his laptop. "It's gone now, Dad. What did the building look like?" As his father described ornate Victorian architecture with pink sandstone corner blocks, Richard's eyes lit up. "I think those stones are the ones I've been saving for a sculpture."

That was how we learned the story of the blocks that became our mailbox base, and of preschool-age Richard's having gone to the bank with his dad, his reward a fruit-flavored sucker.

When Mr. Raymond became bed-bound, Richard helped administer his medications, changed his diapers, and bathed him. Richard sat with his dad for hours, sometimes talking about Salida, sometimes in companionable silence. The night his father died, we stood vigil with Richard's mom and eldest brother, and Mr. Raymond's favorite hospice aide, our hands resting on Mr. Raymond as his life ebbed. Afterward, Richard and I walked outside in the humid night.

I pointed to the glittering Milky Way, that river of stars said to symbolize the journey souls take from this existence to whatever comes next. "There he goes."

Richard took my hand. "Thank you for listening with your heart."

"He loved you, sweetie," I said. "I'm glad you finally made peace."

In early December 2010, after the good news from Dr. Klein, we drove to Denver for a neurosurgery checkup. After another all clear, we headed straight home, racing an incoming snowstorm. We were leaving the city when my phone buzzed. It was Dad: Mom was back in the hospital, her red-blood-cell count dangerously low. I asked if I needed to come. Dad said no, but Mom wanted to talk to me. I pulled off the highway.

"Please come." Mom's voice was faint. "I need you."

My skin crawled. It was the dream.

"I'm scared," she said. "Please come."

I looked west at clouds trailing the high ridges, then turned to Richard. "It's Mom."

He nodded, not surprised. I took a deep breath. I longed with every fiber of my being for home, and normalcy. Regardless of what I wanted, I knew what I needed to do.

"We'll be there as soon as we can," I said.

Richard reached over and wrapped his arms around me. We sat in the car in silence for a long time, watching as snow clouds thickened, obscuring the distant peaks.

That night, we almost lost Mom. It took an emergency team and two pints of blood to stabilize her. "What's her diagnosis?" I asked the resident on rounds the next morning.

He glanced at my parents, and then stepped out into the hall. I followed.

"Failure to thrive."

"Meaning her body is shutting down?"

"Yes." He looked uncomfortable but sympathetic. "I'm sorry."

I looked over his shoulder. Dad sat next to Mom's bed, her pale hand in his, smiling as they listened to the CD I had compiled for her of stories from my long-running *Wild Lives* radio show. A wave of love washed over me. Mom was fading. I couldn't change that. What I could do was prepare them for the inevitable end I could see, even if they could not.

The previous month, Bill had flown in to visit Mom and Dad. Richard and I drove to Denver to join them. Dad was happy to see us; Mom slumped in her wheelchair, silent. I set up the digital photo frame we had loaded with family pictures in hopes of reviving her happy memories. As the images scrolled past, Mom was puzzled at first. Then her smile appeared. "That's us," she said, pointing to a photo of herself and Dad hiking.

"It is," I responded.

Mom lapsed into silence again, and her eyes slid shut. But her smile remained.

Later, after helping Mom into bed and giving her a goodnight kiss, I escaped to the guest apartment down the hall. Bill and Richard were already there.

"You're right," Bill said, as he poured me a glass of wine. "It feels like she's checking out." He was shocked by how much Mom had declined since he had last visited. "Dad can't see it."

"Well," Richard said, "that's not really surprising, is it? His vision is such that he can't see anything, her included, in any detail."

"What he sees is the woman he's loved for so long, as she was before his vision began to go," I said. "It's sweet, in a way."

"When it's not maddening." Bill's voice was dry.

"Yeah," I responded, "that, too."


After hearing Mom's diagnosis, I took a steadying breath. "Does the hospital have a palliative-care team?"

The doctor brightened. "We do. Are you sure they would want that?"

"No," I said. "But I'll work on it."

After I explained palliative, or "comfort," care, Mom and Dad agreed to meet with the team—if I would participate as their advocate. The team couldn't convene until the next day; Richard and I needed to head home before the snowstorm got worse. The social worker offered to patch me in by speakerphone. I looked at Dad.

"Go," he said, waving his hand in dismissal.

"Can we keep the CD?" Mom asked, her voice a whisper. "I'm not finished listening."

"I made it for you, Mom. I love you."

I bent to kiss her cheek. Her hand shook as she reached to stroke my hair, taking me straight back to childhood.

It was a hot July afternoon. We were on day one of a weeklong backpacking trip in California's Sierra Nevada range. I stopped, taking shallow breaths. Mom paused beside me.

"Okay, B-bug?" she asked, stroking my cap of short hair.

"Just catching my breath." On steep trails, I often run out of air, stop until I can breathe again, and then have to hike fast to catch up.

Mom reached into the pocket of her loose denim hiking culottes and pulled out a foil packet containing a cinnamon Pop-Tart, my favorite. My eyes widened. Where had that come from? The night before we'd left, I had watched Mom and her childhood friend Carol carefully weigh and package freeze-dried food for the trip. Pop-Tarts were not included.

I took a bite of the sweet, sticky treat. "How. . ." I started to ask.

Mom put a finger over her lips. "Shh! They're our secret." Her blue eyes danced.

When the palliative-care team recommended that Mom be released into hospice care, my folks were shocked. Dad literally couldn't see how frail Mom was. His mental vision was clouded, too, by his relentlessly optimistic temperament.

"I'm not ready to die," Mom repeated in her faint voice. "I want to go home."

I listened, sympathized, and explained that hospice was Mom's only route home. "Otherwise, you'll have to stay in the hospital."

Silence. Then Dad spoke. "If that's our only option, we'll try it. You'll make the arrangements." It was not a question.

I sighed and reminded myself that while it was frustrating for me to be my parents' caregiver, it was likely equally hard for them to be dependent on me.

Later on the day Mom was discharged, we learned that the hospice provider my parents had selected wouldn't take her until she finished the antibiotics prescribed for her skin sores, a week hence. I was stunned. Dad airily assured me they would be fine. I knew he was wrong: He would have to feed, dress, and bathe Mom and get her to the bathroom all on his own. He had no clue what he was in for. We raced back to Denver, Richard at the wheel.

When we arrived, Dad pelted me with questions. I started a list to ask Callie, the visiting nurse who saw Mom three times a week. Then I fed Mom bites of dinner, fed Dad and Richard, and cleaned the kitchen and bathroom. Afterward, we headed to our motel to collapse.

The next day, Monday, Mom was fretful. She was too weak to sit up without help, and she didn't understand why. I kissed her papery cheek, brushed the silver waves of her hair, and sympathized. It was all I could do.

Later, I explained our dilemma to Callie. "Hospice rules differ about medications," she said carefully, and suggested I call the hospice coordinator from her agency. Hallelujah! That afternoon, Pam, a tall, no-nonsense hospice nurse clad in a black leather Harley-Davidson jacket, knocked on the door. She patiently answered Dad's questions and then examined Mom with gentle thoroughness, pursing her lips at the red-rimmed sores eroding Mom's backside. Pam ordered a hospital bed with a special mattress and requested Sharon, "one of our best," as Mom's daily aide.

That night, Richard fell asleep right away; I curled up next to his warm back, shivering, my muscles aching as if a hammer had pounded me all over. I wasn't sick; the symptoms were simply my body's lifelong response to stress.

I remembered lying on the Danish-modern couch in the living room of my childhood home, my head in Mom's lap. I was five and feverish, my body aching. Mom's hands, which had just played a Bach sonata on the piano, soothed my forehead. She sang softly until I slept.

"Thanks, Mom," I said to the memory, and drifted off.

When we arrived at my folks' the next morning, Dad was getting ready to leave for his exercise class. I asked if Mom had eaten. "No, she's still sleeping."

When Mom woke, I brushed her hair and then fed her some organic blueberry-apple-oat baby food. (Pam had suggested baby food would be easier for Mom to eat and easier for Dad to feed her.) Mindful of Dad's comment "Your mother won't eat baby food," I told her it was a smoothie, a small lie justified when Mom swallowed each spoonful eagerly.

After Dad returned from his class, he helped Mom to the commode and then walked, whistling, into their study. I stayed with Mom. She sat and sat, slumping forward until I was afraid she'd fall off.

"Do you think you're finished?" I asked.

"Yes." Her voice was so faint I could barely hear it. I supported her frail body with one arm and gently wiped.

"Ow!"

"I'm sorry, Mom. There's something stuck." I wiped again and dislodged hard chunks, followed by a gush of softer stuff. Ick. As I carefully cleaned Mom and helped her back to bed, I remembered Richard saying during his dad's hospice care, "Wiping your parent's butt is a milestone no one looks forward to." Roger that. I had no idea how awkward and uncomfortable it would feel—and oddly tender as well.

We never expect to parent our parents, especially not dealing with their shit, metaphorical or literal. And the shift isn't easy: physically, emotionally, or financially. No matter how lovingly intended, such caregiving is complicated by the fact that our parents rarely cede authority; in their minds, we're still their kids, even when we're wiping their butts. If we are fortunate, all concerned will come to a gracious—or at least resigned—acceptance. If not, we will do the best we can. And drink more wine, eat more chocolate, vent to our friends—whatever we need to do to cope. I consumed a lot of chocolate that winter.

Adjusting to new realities is never easy. The challenge is to approach change with an open mind and open heart, and to remember that change is part of our DNA. Our species, all life, was born to change, evolving in response to its flux and flow. We have thrived through convulsive events before, whether global ice ages or wars, pandemics or political upheaval. Humans are amazingly adaptive creatures, in great part because of our ability to love each other and life on this blue planet.

Over lunch, Dad reported that the weather forecast predicted another snowstorm the next day. "You should head home while you can." He added, "We're fine."

Pam was on her way with Sharon, so they really were fine. Home, where we had "only" brain cancer to deal with, sounded heavenly. "Okay. I'll feed Mom, and then we'll hit the road."

As Mom sipped spoonfuls of the "soup" I offered (pureed squash baby food spiced with raspberry vinaigrette salad dressing), I told her we were going home.

"How soon will you be back?" Her frail voice still had spirit. "As in, how many days?"

I chuckled weakly. "Monday."

"That's too long."

"It's less than a week, Mom. We'll be back sooner if you need us."

She closed her eyes. I kissed her forehead. "I love you."

"I love you, too." The words were barely audible.


Dad walked us down to the lobby of their building.

"How long do you think it will be?" he asked abruptly.

Who had appointed me the expert? Richard put his arm around me. "I don't know, Dad."

"I need more time to get used to it."

I saw again Mom's emaciated body and paper-thin skin with ulcerated sores. "A month? Two months?"

"That's okay, then," he said.

"It's not a guarantee, Dad." My voice was sharper than I intended.

"If I just have until . . . oh, mid-January, I think I'll be ready. Do you want to be here when she"—he paused—"dies?"

That, I was sure about. "If I can. I want to hold her hand."

Dad nodded. We hugged him. Then we escaped for home, Richard at the wheel.

*storm clouds muffle peaks*
*snowflakes hiss on wind*
*you sleep, life fading*

# chapter sixteen

*Day Fifteen*

Odometer Reading: 2,689 Miles

After our picnic lunch, we drove to Hawthorne Gallery, south of Big Sur, long a favorite stop for Richard to admire Albert Paley's work. When I parked at the gallery that afternoon, though, his face was sad. "I don't know if I have the energy to go in."

"How about resting on a bench in the sun for a while?" I suggested.

He nodded, pulled himself out of the car, and stretched full-length on a nearby bench, eyes closed. I kissed him. "I'll stay close."

I wandered the garden, shooting photos of fuzzy bumblebees feeding on native bush-lupine flowers and sculptural water features. When I looked back to check on Richard, the bench was empty. Heart racing, I scanned the grounds and then spotted him entering the gallery, a smile on his face. All was well.

That winter of Mom's dying, we settled into a routine of spending three days with my parents and four days at home, recovering. Richard kept up his extreme health regimen and began sketching our plan for the Carpenter Ranch landscape. I read, cooked, and wrote, banking energy for our return to Hospice Central, as I had dubbed my parents' apartment. As the winter solstice approached, we nixed our annual Light the Darkness party again. Now that Mom was fading, we just didn't feel celebratory. "We'll revive the party next year," Richard said. But by the next winter, he was gone. We held the celebration of his life on the winter solstice instead.

On our next trip to Denver, Richard drove us on winding roads whitened by a blanket of fresh snow. At my parents' apartment, he meditated while I sat with Mom. She was fretful and imperious by turns.

"What's wrong?" I asked.

"I'm not ready to go yet." She sounded so annoyed, I had to suppress a chuckle.

"We don't get to decide, Mom. Your body is winding down. I'm sorry."

She cut her blue eyes sideways at me. "I didn't give it permission."

"I know, but remember? You taught us to be gracious with what we can't change."

"I guess so." She sounded pouty, more teenage than a few months shy of eighty years old.

"Richard and I have been working on finding the grace in our time together," I said. "We're not perfect, and we stumble a lot. But our intent is to enjoy our days as best we can."

"You're a good example." Mom's grudging tone made the words less of a compliment.

I plowed on anyway, hoping to help her find peace with the

inevitable. "So are you. You've touched a lot of people in your life." I reminded her of the schools where she had worked, the birding and nature workshops she and Dad had taught, the national parks and other places where they had volunteered. "You've made a difference."

Mom was quiet. "I love you," she finally said, and closed her eyes.

On the weekly commute in mid-January, I relaxed while Richard drove. Cocooned in the car, with snow swirling around us, I could almost forget we were headed to the city to "midwife" Mom's dying, a term Richard first used to describe easing his dad's transition. We think of midwifing only for birth, but "bring something into being" can also refer to freeing spirit from body in death, a process just as laborious and unavoidable.

"The bright spot for me these days," I said, "is that we're working together again and you're engaged in your art."

"So, from your perspective, I'm back." Richard slowed for a stretch of black ice.

I thought. "It seems to me it's more than just being 'back.' I'd say you've rewoven severed connections, the way I darn a hole in a sock by weaving new threads over it. The hole remains, but the darning restores the fabric of the sock."

Richard smiled. "I like that metaphor. I'm reweaving brain connections lost to the tumors. Thank you." He took my hand as we sped between dazzling snowbanks under blue sky.

In Denver, Dad was happy to see us; Mom was curled in a fetal position on the bed. I straightened her, adjusted her pillows, and then fixed dinner for Dad and Richard. As I fed Mom bites of Richard's sourdough bread soaked in baby-food "soup," I recalled Richard's suggestion that finding happy memories might assuage her Alzheimer's-induced anxiety.

"Did you and Granddaddy Milner go camping when you were a kid?" I asked.

"Yes." Her voice was barely audible. A smile drifted across her face.

"Do you remember how old you were when you first went camping?"

"Before high school." I had to lean close to hear her.

"Where did you go?"

"Yosemite." The smile grew. "Tuolumne Meadows."

I could imagine that much younger Mom, tall and strong, hiking mountain trails with her dad, wavy brunette hair blowing in the breeze.

"Thanks for sharing the wild with us," I said, as she drifted into sleep, still smiling.

Dad called as Richard and I ate breakfast at our hotel the next morning. Mom had gotten out of bed sometime before dawn, fallen, and lain on the carpet until Dad had found her. They were at the hospital, waiting for scans.

"Don't hurry," Dad said. "Finish your breakfast."

We raced across the city and found our way to the ER just in time to hear the news: Mom's hip was broken. Her paper-thin bones and eroding sores made successful repair unlikely. The orthopedic surgeon—a slender, serious-faced woman—spoke directly to Mom. "There's nothing solid to anchor to. Any hardware we install would invite further infection."

Mom was scared but lucid. She shook her head. "No surgery. I want to go home."

"Do you understand you won't be able to walk?"

"I know."

The surgeon looked at us. "Are you okay with that?" We three nodded.

The hospital released Mom to a rehabilitation facility. When we arrived at the place, I swallowed dismay. The exterior was dingy cement blocks with small windows—more jail than rehab. Inside, Mom's room shocked me: It was shabby, bare but for the hospital bed she lay in. A smartly dressed woman was pressing Dad to sign a stack of forms. I interrupted to ask about furniture.

"We're bringing things. He needs to sign these forms."

"He's legally blind," I said sweetly, invoking the Americans with Disabilities Act.

She glared at me.

"Dad, do you want me to read the forms for you?" He nodded, suppressing a grin.

She tapped her foot while I read.

Later, I called Natalie, Richard's social worker at the VA, and described Mom's situation. "What should we do?"

"Call the hospice coordinator. Tell them you want an evaluation. Ask them to meet y'all at the rehab center to discuss options. And call me if you need support."

I exhaled. "You're the best. Thank you."

The next morning, the hospice staff met us in Mom's room, where Dad had slept in a recliner next to her bed. They asked

Mom how she was. "Fine," she said, her voice faint but firm. "And I want to go home."

I stifled a chuckle. Mom couldn't sit up, and her mind wasn't always clear, but she could still sound commanding.

The hospice team conferred and decided that if we could arrange in-home, twenty-four-hour care, Mom could be released. I began making calls. By two o'clock, I had everything set up: Mom and Dad would be home by dinnertime, with caregivers in place. If we left right away, Richard and I could make it over the mountains before dark. I asked Dad if that was okay.

"Absolutely." He waved his hand dismissively. "We're set."

Hardly. But I had done what I could. I hugged Mom. "You'll be home soon."

"Thank you, Suz." Her voice was barely audible. "I love you."

"I love you, too, Mom."

"Good work," Richard said, as he climbed into the driver's seat of the car.

"No way was I going to leave Mom in that place." I reached for his hand and closed my eyes, letting the adrenaline that had carried me through advocating for Mom drain out of my body. "Thanks for driving. I'm wrung out."

"That's what you have me for," Richard said lightly. "We'll be home tonight, and we'll work together to get rested up for the next trip." He sounded so like the prelobectomy Richard, compassionate and capable, that my eyes filled with tears. *All will be well,* I thought.


At Hawthorne Gallery, Richard studied the flowing steel base of an Albert Paley table. I was reminded of the first sink he sculpted.

He had just begun exploring terraphilia, and what local rocks have to teach us about the earth.

He chose a weathered gneiss boulder, roughly the size of a flattened basketball, "foraged" from a road cut in western Colorado. Pink feldspar veins zigzagged through a charcoal-gray matrix flecked with sparkling mica. He perched the boulder on a counter in his shop and studied it until he could visualize the basin inside, and then began carving and polishing. The afternoon he finished, he called me: "Come see!" I walked over to his studio. Richard beamed as he cradled the sixty-pound rock like a baby in his arms. The exterior was still rough; the highly polished oval basin revealed the beauty inside the rock. "It worked!" he said, his voice drenched in wonder.

The memory gave me an idea. I wandered out to the deck of the gallery and stared at the distant ocean. At a stone-carving workshop Richard had taught, Grant Pound, executive director of Colorado Art Ranch and a personal friend, had commented that he'd like to apprentice with Richard. Teaching Grant, I thought, might breathe life into my love's inner artist.

In the car later, I reminded Richard of Grant's comment. "Would you be interested in taking him on as an apprentice? It would be a way of passing on your sculpture aesthetic." I didn't say *before you die.* We both understood that.

Richard said slowly, "I could do that." He handed me his phone. I dialed Grant's number and handed it back. By the time we were aimed south on Highway 1, I heard Grant's enthusiastic "When do we start?"

Richard's smile grew as they made plans. "Thanks for giving me something to look forward to," he said after the call, and closed his eyes, still smiling.

The last day of January, we were back at Hospice Central, where the weather was bitterly cold. A high of one degree Fahrenheit did not daunt Bill and Dad, who were headed out to look for an out-of-range curve-billed thrasher, a desert species Dad had studied when the kids lived in Tucson. "The poor bird is probably frozen." I rooted in the closet for Dad's warmest parka.

"I just hope I can see it." He carefully wiped his binocular lenses. The motion reminded me of Dad's adjusting his binoculars for my six-year-old face one winter day in Florida and then aiming my gaze and the lenses toward a scrub-jay. I had gasped at the sparkle in those black eyes, each blue feather crisp. I still feel the thrill, and the intimacy, of that view.

"Me too." I hugged Dad.

After the birders left, Richard meditated while I sat with Mom. She had quit eating and rarely spoke, but she seemed content to just be.

Dad and Bill returned at lunchtime, red-faced and half-frozen but jubilant: They had seen the thrasher. They recounted their adventures while slurping my homemade tortellini soup.

When Pam arrived, she was shocked by the change in Mom's condition. She texted the hospice physician and then called a family meeting in the living room.

"It won't be long." Pam focused on each of us in turn. "Probably not tomorrow, but soon. Are you all okay with that?"

We nodded.

"She's struggling still. Each of you needs to let her know it's okay to let go."

Richard, Bill, and I turned as one to look at Dad.

"We've each talked to her, Dad," I said. "Have you?"

He hemmed and hawed and finally said they had "talked around it."

Pam looked at him. "I know you don't want Joan to suffer. You need to talk with her."

Cornered, Dad nodded. "I will."

Words matter. We've all heard stories about patients who will themselves to hang on, worried about leaving those they love. And then once they hear it's okay to let go, they do—sometimes within minutes. Death is as normal as birth. It is time to acknowledge that passage not as a failure, but as an integral part of life. Loss hurts, but we make death more difficult by resisting the reality that all lives end—sooner or later. With our endings come the potential for new beginnings, as the circles and cycles of life itself continue on.

Pam left, Bill headed to the airport for his flight home, Dad immersed himself in his birding files, and Richard strode the halls of the apartment building for exercise. I sat with Mom, holding her cold hand in mine as she dozed.

That evening, Dad asked in a worried tone, "Are you planning on going home tomorrow?"

"No," I said. "We're here for the duration."


Two days later, our friend Peg visited with her four-year-old daughter, Mariela.

"Hello, Peg. Hello, Mariela." Mom spoke for the first time in several days, startling me.

Mariela crawled up on the bed and gave Mom a careful hug. "I love you, Joan."

Mom smiled and dozed again. Peg sang to Mom in her sweet soprano voice; Mariela went to the living room to read with Dad; I wrote in my journal.

When Pam arrived, she checked on Mom and then took me into the kitchen, where she pulled the box labeled "Comfort Kit" out of the fridge. "You're the one who will most likely be using this," she said, as she explained each drug. Then she headed off to tend to a dying patient across town. "If anything happens, call me."

I was in the kitchen when Peg called, "Suz!"

I raced to the bedroom. Mom was trying to sit up, grimacing in pain. I checked the clock: almost time for her next dose of painkillers. I powdered a tablet with a little liquid, sucked the resultant slurry into a syringe—a trick Pam had shown me—squirted it into Mom's mouth, and wiped her forehead. She relaxed. Fifteen minutes later, though, she began sweating and reared up again. I called Pam.

"Give her another dose of oxycodone. Call back in fifteen minutes if it doesn't help."

It didn't. An agonizing half hour, two more calls to Pam, and two drugs from the hospice comfort kit passed before Mom quit sweating and opened her eyes. Peg and I sponged her face; Richard helped me replace her soaked pillowcase and reposition her in bed.

The crisis past, Peg brought Mariela in to say goodbye. Mom held Peg's hand and smiled.

That smile remained for the rest of the evening. When Richard told a joke, Mom raised her eyebrows and slid her gaze his way. I reminded her of the time Bill and I had tried to sneak a gallon jar of tadpoles home from a weekend trip. The jar tipped over when Dad braked suddenly, flooding the camper with pond water and slippery, wriggling creatures.

Mom smiled and made her nose twitch like a rabbit, a trick I had forgotten.

At dinnertime, Dad and Richard went to the dining room. I sat with Mom. When they returned, she opened her eyes with a puzzled look. "It's me, Mom. Suz." I squeezed her hand. She smiled. Dad hummed enthusiastically in the kitchen. Mom moved her eyes that way, smiled, and then looked back at me with raised eyebrows.

"That's Dad, humming in the kitchen—at least he's on key for a change."

Her smile grew. She shut her eyes.

At seven, I gave Mom her nighttime meds and kissed her cheek. "Don't forget that I love you." Richard kissed her other cheek. "Good night, Joan." She opened her eyes and smiled.

Richard and I walked hand in hand down the hall to the guest apartment to decompress. Just before we went to bed, I checked on Mom. She was sleeping; Dad was brushing his teeth.

My phone buzzed at 7:03 the next morning. It was Dad. "I think Joan's gone."

I woke Richard and raced down the hall. Dad was in the kitchen, carefully pouring himself a glass of orange juice, one eye shut to focus better. "When I woke just now, I thought Joan said something. But when I checked, she wasn't breathing."

In the bedroom, Mom was still. I lifted one wrist: warm, no pulse. I kissed her forehead and called Pam. Then I shooed Dad and Richard, still groggy, to the dining room for breakfast.

I sat with Mom and thought about her life: The wavy-haired, blue-eyed college student who met Dad at the University of California, a six-block walk from her childhood home, and made him wait until she graduated to get married. Who earned a master's degree in library science—cum laude—despite being legally blind. Mom, whose smile lit up a room; who prized birdsong, wildflowers, and mountain hikes as much as chocolate. Who had fought letting go and then found the grace to lead the way on her final trail.

Snow began to trickle from the gray sky. I looked at the calendar: It was two months to the day before Mom's eightieth birthday. I wiped away tears, grief mixed with relief that she had died so peacefully—and, although this may sound selfish, that I would no longer be pulled between her care and Richard's needs.

"Bye, Mom," I said aloud in the silence. "I miss you."


As the months passed and brain cancer again consumed our days, I occasionally heard Mom's voice singing softly, the way she used to sing us to sleep, and I smiled, the grief almost sweet.

*snow falls*
*heart stilled, songs quiet*
*winter settles in*

# chapter seventeen

*Day Fifteen*

Odometer Reading: 2,701 Miles

It was late afternoon by the time I aimed the car down the steep driveway leading to the cabins strung along the cliff at Lucia Lodge, a historic inn built in the 1930s to serve travelers on newly opened Highway 1. Our cabin overlooked the cove far below, and miles of wild coast. It is a magical spot; we once watched a gray whale swim through the cove without surfacing and vanish around the point, the barnacles patterning its huge body perfectly clear.

Evening fog crept in as I ferried our gear to the cabin, with its weathered aqua-blue shutters. Richard settled into an Adirondack chair out front. After unpacking, I joined him, bearing his Belgian ale and my sparkling water. Wrapped in his brown pile hoodie, the fuchsia hedge behind him blooming with crimson stars, Richard smiled and raised his glass to me. "This feels like a real honeymoon." It did.

The week before Mom died, we returned to the VA for Richard's January checkup. He proudly handed Dr. Klein the loaf of crusty whole-wheat boule he had baked for her, along with a container of his sourdough starter. She sniffed appreciatively and smiled. "You're baking again. How are you feeling?"

"Watch." He took his juggling balls out of his briefcase and tossed them into the air overhand. She laughed. He raised one foot, still juggling.

She applauded and then said that his latest MRI looked clear, except for "increasing nodularity" in the tissue around where his tumors had been removed. "It may be nothing," she said, "but we're going to watch it. You're clearly healthy," she added. "That's a good sign."

Back at home the next night, I cooked one of Richard's favorite meals: eggs baked on spinach, topped with my green chile sauce. He ate with gusto. For dessert, I dished up bowls of Cherry Garcia ice cream with a splash of port. Later, we made leisurely love, reclaiming our good life. *All will be well.*

After Mom's death, we stayed in Denver for a few days to help Dad. Richard, so present at that appointment with Dr. Klein, was now groggy and slow. "It's a sinus infection," he said. I didn't question his conclusion.

In the car heading home, Richard closed his eyes. "I have a headache."

A chill skittered across my skin. "How much on the pain scale?"

"Two, maybe three."

"Should I turn around? We can be at the VA hospital in twenty minutes."

He thought for a moment. "No, it's just my sinuses. We both need home and rest."

My intuition said I should turn around. I hesitated and then pressed on, exhausted.

That decision haunts me. Could I have prevented what was to come? I don't know. The truth is, after midwifing Mom's death, I was out of gas. I didn't want to see that something was wrong. That's human: When the truth is too overwhelming, too huge, too impossible to deal with, sometimes we simply can't face it.

At home, Richard was better some days, foggier on others. One morning, I visited a friend's middle-school class to talk about writing and returned home to find the guy who three weeks earlier had baked perfect loaves of sourdough boule now unable to manage a simple batch of biscuits. The kitchen was covered in flour; bowls and utensils were scattered everywhere. He was standing amid the chaos, confused. I swore silently, took a deep breath, got Richard and the biscuits back on track, and cleaned up.

Saturday morning, almost a week after we returned, Richard woke himself for the first time since Mom had died, took his meds, wrote them in his chart, came back to bed, and pulled me close. "I've been pretty out of it. You must be exhausted. What can I do for you?"

I burst into tears. He was back!

Richard fetched tissues and kissed me, and then rubbed my back until I was so relaxed that we slipped into lovemaking. Afterward, we snuggled close, skin to skin. He fell back to sleep. I got up, did yoga, and went to the kitchen to make breakfast, profoundly grateful to have my partner back.

It didn't last. When Richard woke, his brain was foggy again. It took him two hours to eat breakfast. At noon, he reported that his headache pain was a six. "I'm going to take a nap." When I couldn't rouse him later, I panicked and called our family doctor at home. I explained the headache and grogginess. Mary didn't hesitate. "Get Richard to the ER now! I'll brief Dr. Adams, the doctor on shift there."

"Okay." I gulped back tears. "Thank you."

I raced into our bedroom and shook Richard. "Mary says I need to take you to the ER."

"Okay." His voice was slurred. He pushed himself to his feet and staggered. I caught him and somehow directed his wobbling steps out the back door, along the porch, and into the garage. I balanced his weight with one hip and wrenched the car door open. He slid into the seat as if boneless. By the time I got the car started, his eyes had closed again.

"Stay with me, sweetie, okay?"

"I'm with you," he mumbled.

At the emergency room entrance, I rushed around and opened Richard's door. His eyes were closed.

"Stay there. I'll get a wheelchair." I dashed inside.

A nurse helped me wheel Richard into an exam room and got him onto the table. I held his hand. She checked his vitals: His pulse was dangerously high, his blood pressure low.

"Stay with me, sweetie."

"I'm here." His voice dragged.

Dr. Adams ordered a scan of Richard's brain. The minutes crawled. I held his hand and talked to him. Finally, Dr. Adams returned and pointed to an image on the screen of the computer he had wheeled in: "See the fluid accumulation?"

Richard closed his eyes. I felt sick. Fluid was compressing his right brain laterally and also pushing it down on the brain stem.

Why hadn't I taken him directly to the VA hospital, instead of home? I swallowed.

"We need to get him to Denver as soon as we can," Dr. Adams said. He left to make calls.

A few minutes later, my phone buzzed. It was Bill. I told him the news.

"Damn. Do you want me to fly to Denver and meet you?"

I gulped. "No, but thank you. I'll keep you posted."

"Tell Richard to hang in there. I want to take him out birding." I relayed the message.

"Other jays." Richard's slow words alluded to a birding trick my brother had played on him decades before.

Bill laughed. "He's still with us. Hang in there. I love you."

I swallowed tears and called Molly. No answer. I called Kerry and Dave.

"We'll drive you to Denver," Kerry said immediately. "Go home and gather what you need. We'll pick you up there."

I tried to think and couldn't. Richard's eyes were closed, but he was breathing. "Okay."


The dashboard clock read 11:07 when Dave pulled onto the highway. Kerry was in the passenger seat; I sat in the backseat with Little, their cattle dog. The red taillights of the ambulance shone ahead of us. We talked for a while, high on adrenaline, and then fell silent. The highway wound into darkness beyond the cone of the headlights. My Richard mantra spun in my mind like a prayer wheel in the wind: *Healthy brain. Healthy body. Heathy heart. Healthy spirit. Healthy Richard . . .*

It was past two thirty by the time Dave stopped the truck at the front entrance of the VA hospital. "Do you want us to come in?"

"No, thanks. I know where to go."

"Call us," Kerry said. "We won't drive home until we hear from you."

I nodded and patted a sleepy Little. "Thank you."

The hospital atrium was eerily quiet. I took an elevator to the fourth floor. In the ICU, Richard, eyes closed, was answering questions from the head Neurosurgery resident.

"What kind of building is this?" Dr. Shaefer asked.

The answer was slurred and slow but vintage Richard: "Structurally or functionally? Functionally, it's a hospital. Structurally, I don't know."

I laughed with relief—he was still there!—and teased Richard about being a smart-ass.

After Dr. Shaefer left, I curled up in an armchair next to Richard's bed and conked out.

When I woke a few hours later, Richard was out of bed, hospital gown askew. "What's wrong, sweetie?"

"I have to pee. Where's the urinal?"

As I looked around, he squatted on the floor.

"You can't pee there!"

I dashed out to find his night nurse. By the time I returned, Richard was back in bed, asleep. A puddle of yellow urine spread across the floor.

"I'm sorry," I said, embarrassed. "He's not usually like this."

"I've seen a lot worse." She smiled reassuringly and fetched a mop.

At midmorning that next day, we learned that the neurosurgery team planned to drill into Richard's skull to release cranial fluid dammed by a blood clot and thus relieve the pressure on his brain. The surgery could be done right in his ICU room but required a blood transfusion.

"Before you consent," Dr. Shaefer said, "you need to know that the odds of getting a blood-borne disease from a transfusion are one in two million."

"That's better odds than the lottery." Richard's slow voice was amused.

I laughed. A grin creased Dr. Shaefer's round face.

Two hours later, Richard sat up in bed, eyes open, talking normally. He smiled broadly when I entered the room. "There's my sweetie!" A threaded, chrome-plated nozzle stuck out of his skull just above the ridge of his lobectomy scar, draining into a suction pouch. It looked creepy. But he was back.

I snapped a photo and texted it to Molly. His phone buzzed. "Great head jewelry," I heard Molly say. "Very Lady Gaga–ish."

Richard, immune to pop culture, looked puzzled. I chuckled. "I'll explain later."

When I did, Richard said, "I don't remember getting here. Did I miss Joan's memorial?"

I recounted the story and then reassured him that Mom's memorial was still a week away.

"I should be released by then," he said. "I can help."

"I can use your help. For now, let's just focus on your recovery."

The day after Richard's drain procedure was Valentine's Day. For the first time in our twenty-eight years together, there was no freshly baked cheesecake, no snuggling in bed, no lovemaking. At least he was with us, I reminded myself.

After my morning walk, I returned to his ICU room to find two visitors sitting on folding stools by his bed. The woman, tall, with streaky blond hair, smiled and stood up. "I'm Elizabeth Holman, psychologist with the palliative-care team, and this is Scott de la Cruz, a resident."

"We don't need palliative care," I said, panic in my voice. I had just lost Mom. I could not—would not—consider losing Richard. I took a breath, searching for graciousness. "We had palliative care for my mom. It was a gift."

Elizabeth looked sympathetic. "Richard was telling us about that. I'm so sorry for your loss. Let's just say we're here to help coordinate Richard's care."

They resumed discussing Richard's medical living will form.

"I want to allow my team maximum flexibility as long as treatment has a reasonable expectation of extending my life in healthy ways," he said. "I also want to make it clear that when intervention no longer makes sense from a quality-of-life perspective, I want to be allowed to die gracefully."

"Wow." Elizabeth smiled. "I wish all our patients were so thoughtful and articulate."

Richard looked at me. "Suz, can you write that down? I'm afraid I won't remember it."

I opened my laptop, hoping fervently we wouldn't need those words anytime soon.

Four days after that terrifying night ride over the mountains, Richard was released from the hospital—sans Lady Gaga head jewelry. In our Denver motel room that night, he carefully put toothpaste on his toothbrush and then asked, "Do you still want to do the Pacific coast trip next month?"

Before the holidays, a group of friends had surprised us with a check "for the honeymoon you never got to take." Stunned and grateful, we decided to drive the Pacific coast, our favorite ocean edge. Then came Mom's decline. Now, I ached for time away. "If you're up for it."

"I think we both need the break," Richard said.

"Let's do it."

I woke later to the creak of the motel-room door opening. Richard was headed out into the snowy night. "Sweetie, where are you going?" I kept my voice calm, with an effort.

"To the bathroom." He sounded annoyed, as if it were obvious.

"It's the other way." I groped for the light switch. Richard stood in the doorway in his pajama bottoms, barefoot, gripping his crotch. I herded him to the bathroom just in time.

Back in bed later, he pulled me close. "I didn't mean to scare you. I was just confused."

"I know, sweetie. It's okay." He snuggled his long body next to mine and fell back to sleep. I lay awake, haunted by the image of my brilliant but clearly still impaired love silhouetted in the dark doorway. What if I hadn't woken? I didn't want to imagine him lost or, worse, in a strange place. Clearly, this wasn't the time to take our honeymoon trip. I felt tears rise and pushed them back, reminding myself of a Buddhist saying Richard often quoted: "Pain is inevitable, suffering optional." I deliberately breathed out suffering.

We still had each other. We would go home after Mom's memorial service. Richard would heal. With that thought, I fell asleep.

A week later, we were back at home in Salida. Richard built a fire in the woodstove while I unpacked. Dave and Kerry knocked on the door, bearing a dinner tray with fragrant quiche, freshly tossed salad, and warm oatmeal cookies.

After we ate, Richard eyed the skylight above our bed. Its light-blocking blind dangled, cord broken.

"Don't worry about the blind, sweetie," I said. "It'll keep."

"I think I know how to fix it. It won't take long." He grinned, face mischievous. "Of course, that's what I always say." He laughed and went out to his studio. He returned carrying a nine-foot-tall ladder, his big cordless drill, and some hardware and nylon cord.

"Are you sure you're okay on the ladder?" A week before, he hadn't been able to stand without help.

"Neurosurgery didn't say anything about not climbing ladders," he said, voice confident. *Because it didn't occur to them that you would try*, I thought. He climbed to the very top step and sat down. I headed to the kitchen, unable to watch. The whine of the drill drew me back. Richard threaded the cord through a small pulley now attached to the lower corner of the skylight. "Pull the cord."

I did. The blind unrolled smoothly. "You're magic."

He grinned from his perch. "Apparently, my right brain is back."

All *would* be well.

*spooned in bed*
*stars wheel in night sky*
*spring sprouts in our hearts*

## chapter eighteen

❦

## Day Fifteen

### Evening

At Lucia Lodge, we climbed into the four-poster bed under a comforter as thick as the fog bank muffling the ocean outside. Richard pulled me close. "My brain wants to make love, but my body isn't listening. Will you take a rain check? Or a brain check?" He chuckled. "Or a . . . I can't think of another word."

"Brain drain?" I suggested, and that made him laugh again, the sound vibrating deep in his chest. He had always loved words and word play. He regularly consulted my two-volume *Oxford English Dictionary* for just the right word—a skill that helped him excel as an expert witness. Now he was losing words as he lost control of his body, the muscular form he had always used so proudly and so well.

In the six weeks after his brain-drain surgery, Richard came close to death twice more because of fluid accumulation and recovered miraculously each time. The next two crises required his neuro-surgery team to reopen the Zipper and remove his skull plate to undam the flow. The first time came just eight days after we returned home from the drain procedure, when Richard announced at lunchtime that he had a headache. I asked what his pain level was.

"Five," he said, voice slow.

*Hell.* I drove him directly to the emergency room, where, luckily for us, Dr. Adams was on duty. He congratulated Richard on how great he looked and ordered a CT scan. When Dr. Adams showed us the images, Richard, who had no memory of the previous scan, was impressed at the volume of fluid again compressing his right brain. I was shocked and scared.

"I'm going to get started on transferring you to the VA hospital," Dr. Adams said.

"Can I drive him?" I asked.

Dr. Adams smiled. "If Richard agrees."

Richard laughed. "I'm going to remember the trip this time."

It was dusk by the time we set out, and the roads were icy. Richard dozed most of the way. But at the VA hospital, he awakened, slung his briefcase over his shoulder, and grabbed our suitcase. We walked up the stairs, and he strode through the doors at the ICU. "I'm Richard Cabe, and I understand you have a bed for me," he announced, and then recited his identification number.

The nurse at the desk stared—and then smiled. "I don't think we've ever had a patient walk in under their own power before," she said, as she checked him in.

By the next morning, he was sinking again. When Dr. Brega stopped by to let us know his surgery was scheduled for the following day, I voiced concern about how much Richard's alertness and brain function had deteriorated since just the night before.

Dr. Brega looked thoughtful. "The problem is finding OR

time and assembling my team." She added, "I'm a single mom, and I try not to schedule work at night, so I can be home for my ten-year-old son. Fourth-grade homework is harder than you think—especially math."

Richard laughed and then said, his words slow, "When I recover, I'll tutor him."

"I'll hold you to that," Dr. Brega responded. She walked to the whiteboard and picked up a marker. "Here is what we see." She drew a cross-section of the skull and brain and added a line around the inside of the skull for the dura, the membrane lining. Then she drew a flattened oval, a hematoma, in the space between the brain and the dura. "Because a hematoma is rich in proteins, when a membrane forms around it, fluid flows into it from the surrounding tissue—"

"Osmotic pressure," Richard croaked, his left brain clearly still working.

She smiled. "Exactly. The membrane is vascularized, so we would rather not remove it and potentially add more sources of bleeding. We think the hematoma itself has caused irritation. We'll know more tomorrow when we open your skull plate."

An hour later, Dr. Brega was back with the news that she had "bumped up" Richard's surgery to that very evening after looking at his latest CT scan.

"Who will do it?" I asked, concerned.

"I will. My nanny will pick up my son from school, and my mother will babysit."

"Thank you." Richard's eyes were closed, his voice halting.

She smiled. "You just saved me from fourth-grade math."

Fourth grade was a fraught time for Molly. She was living with her mom during school years, with us in summers. That June, we took her to Arkansas for her cousin Carolyn's high school graduation. Molly was her sunny self for the whole trip, happily soaking up family stories and playing cards with her cousins, aunt, and grandparents—until the day we were to leave.

After breakfast, Carolyn sought me out. "Suz, I'm worried about Molly."

"What's wrong?"

"She says she doesn't want to go back to Colorado."

"Oh," I said. This was familiar, and sad. "Thanks for letting me know."

I fetched Richard. Molly, face mutinous, was sitting on Carolyn's bed, kicking the frame.

"What's wrong, sweetie?" Richard asked.

"I want to live with you guys. I've lived with Mom for long enough. It's your turn!" She burst into tears. I put my arm around her; Richard snuggled her from her other side. We regarded each other over her dark head. The custody arrangement was not in our favor. But Molly's unhappiness decided me. It was time to push for change.

"We'll make it happen, sweetie," I said. Richard looked surprised. "I promise."

A few months later, Molly injured her foot so badly she couldn't walk. We flew her to Iowa, where we lived then, for specialized care. After a few weeks with us, she was skipping again. Her mother grudgingly agreed that Molly could stay for the rest of the semester. The adjustment was not smooth, and more than once I wondered why I was so sure we'd make it work. Yet somehow we did, and that summer, Molly's temporary move became permanent.

Two afternoons after Richard's surgery, Matt, Richard's ICU nurse, helped me move him to a single room in the newly renovated palliative-care ward. We exclaimed over the plank floor, the soft lighting, the stylish recliner chair, and the bath, more like a hotel room than a hospital.

After Matt left, Richard patted the bed and grinned. "We could see if it works."

I smiled, exhausted but charmed. "The door doesn't lock, sweetie. But I'm glad you're back, and in the mood."

"It'll wait until we get home," he said, voice confident.


Sunday morning, Richard was discharged, the Zipper freshly stapled. I drove us across the city to visit Dad on the way home. As I sorted Dad's mail and Richard rested, Dad mentioned that he was considering moving. My hands stopped. I couldn't imagine managing his move right then.

"Just to a smaller apartment within the building," Dad added quickly. "I won't need your help. I'll hire Monique [one of Mom's caregivers] to pack and movers for the furniture."

"Okay, Dad." I rolled my eyes. Richard, reclining, grinned.


At home, Richard designed and built a sculptural gate to keep the deer out of the kitchen garden, practiced juggling, meditated, and caught up on art-business accounting. He had good days and bad days, good moods and bad moods, but overall he seemed more himself again. But then one Sunday afternoon I watched my brilliant guy get frustrated as he struggled to decipher a phone number on a medical bill. *It's just a bad brain day*, I thought, reluctant to face the implications of another crisis.

Monday morning, two weeks after we had returned home, it took Richard three hours to eat breakfast. When he finished, I drove him directly to the VA medical center in Denver.

"At least we have daylight and the roads are clear," he said.

A stream of hospital staff stopped in to see him, including Elizabeth Holman and Dr. Klein, who watched as Richard juggled and missed catching the balls the nurse had improvised out of bandages. He laughed; Dr. Klein's face was sad. His team put Richard back on steroids, the cranky drugs, to relieve the fluid pressure.

By the next morning, he was much more alert. When Dr. Brega explained the plan to open his skull plate and install a permanent shunt to drain the excess fluid into his peritoneal cavity, he asked whether the magnets in the MRI machine could alter the shunt's settings. I would never have thought of that—and my brain wasn't impaired.

"Theoretically, no; if anything goes wrong, we have a remote to reset the valves."

"Can I borrow it if I need to keep him in line?" I asked. Richard's laugh lifted my spirits.


At five thirty the next morning, my phone buzzed. "I hope I didn't wake you," Richard said. "I just wanted to tell you that I love you before they take me off to surgery. I've said my intentions, and I'm feeling strong and whole."

"I love you, too. I'll be there when you get to the ICU."

Tears ran down my face as I hung up. He was headed for his

fourth craniotomy in eighteen months, his second brain surgery in just thirty days. How much more could he take? How much could I take? I didn't know. I did know that I loved him and was determined that we would make it through this.

Since I was awake, I got up in the dark and began my morning yoga routine, practicing calm and balance in hopes of becoming what I practiced. Sometimes all we can do in the face of crises is to continue our everyday routine. To simply keep living, with as much composure as we can summon.

When Dr. Brega entered the surgery waiting room at noon, her smile was satisfied. "I think we got it this time," she said. The fluid was too thick for a shunt or for another drain. So they had gone to plan C and carefully removed the hematoma. "It's possible it got this thick as a healing response. He's an 'überhealer.' He astonishes us all with how quickly he recovers."

He was already asking for me, she said. "He wakes up like a bear." Dr. Brega shook her head affectionately. "He's so bright. His mind fights to come out of the anesthesia."

Richard smiled when he saw me in the doorway of his ICU room. His head was wrapped in a tidy gauze turban; his voice was hoarse from the breathing tube they had used during surgery.

"There's my love! What's coming out of my skull next to the Zipper?"

"You have two drains, one for the subdural space and one for the incision site," I said. "You can sit up as soon as you feel like it."

I leaned over to kiss him and then sat down, overcome by the usual nausea at seeing him after surgery. Richard was clearly making an effort to be cheerful, but his pain was palpable. I relayed Dr. Brega's report, including her "überhealer" comment. That elicited a smile.

By the time his dinner tray appeared, Richard, only five hours post–brain surgery, was sitting up and eager to eat. As I walked to Starbucks to fetch my own dinner, I heard hope singing again. Richard seemed more "there" than he had since Mom's death. I couldn't articulate exactly what was different, but it was positive. I searched my memory. Then I realized: It was his eye movements. That winter, Richard had begun to stare, his gaze seeming to get stuck. "Don't stare, sweetie. It's not polite," I would remind him. He would wrench his eyes away with an effort I could almost feel, and then his gaze would stick again on whatever it hit next. It was as if his "seeing" had slowed to a crawl. Now his eye movements were quick again, normal.

On Friday evening, when Molly arrived for the weekend, she noticed, too. "He seems more like Dad than he has in a while."

She was right. It wasn't just his vision. Richard was more responsive, and, despite some crankiness from the steroids, more present and empathetic. Hope's song swelled.

Eight days after I drove Richard to Denver for this latest crisis, he signed himself out of the ward, thanked the staff, and led the way confidently down the stairs and out through the warren of halls. (Molly had flown home to San Francisco the afternoon before.)

"You're navigating again," I said, delighted.

"I am, aren't I?" He grinned.

Outside, Richard slipped on his sunglasses against the glare, but his eyes remained wide open, drinking in the view: the robin that darted out of a grove of crabapple trees; the crow perched on the furrowed black branch of an American elm tree; the clarity of a spring-blue sky.

"Wow!" he exclaimed.

"'Wow,' as in the world is richer and more detailed than you remembered?"

"Yes, I had forgotten. It's amazing and wonderful, as in literally full of wonder."

Later, Dr. Brega explained: Each time the fluid accumulated and the pressure increased, Richard's brain triaged tasks, allocating the processing power to the critical ones (breathing and heartbeat, for instance) and slowing all else. Visual processing was one of the first to be choked down—hence the staring. Now, he could see in real time again.

After soaking in the wealth of detail we get used to ignoring, Richard shut his eyes and rested—but only briefly. When I looked over again, he gazed around, face enraptured. *How much we take for granted*, I thought, profoundly grateful to have the chance to see the world through Richard's "new eyes," or, more correctly, his revived right brain. That renewed view of everyday marvels was a gift, and also a reminder that even in the most difficult times, there are moments worth savoring.

After dinner that night, we watched a sliver of new moon, magnified by the layer of city air pollution, set behind the distant peaks of the Front Range.

"Wow!" Richard exclaimed again, and pulled me close for a kiss.

Later, he sat on the bed in our motel room, reading glasses on, carefully cutting paper and cardboard and forming them into curvilinear mock-ups of wall sculptures he imagined fabricating with galvanized sheet steel. The shapes undulated like the mountain ridges at home. Watching him work, I sent a prayer of thanksgiving to the universe.

Richard truly was back. All *would* be well.

*silver crescent*
*April moon glimmers anew*
*clear as your eyes*

# chapter nineteen

## Day Fifteen

### Night

As darkness fell, fog enveloped our cabin at Lucia Lodge, muffling even the crash of the waves on the rocks far below. We fell asleep in deep quiet. Around 4:00 a.m., I woke to Richard's snoring and realized he was sweaty. I pulled back the comforter, and he quieted. I lay awake, conscious of a new noise: I could hear the waves again.

I slid from bed and padded out the door in bare feet. The fog had sunk below the cliff; stars dazzled the entire bowl of sky. I dashed inside and woke Richard. "The fog dropped. Come see the stars!"

I guided him out the door and down the dark steps. He turned his gaze upward.

"Oh!" His slow voice breathed awe. "Thank you for showing me."

Five months earlier, less than twenty-four hours after Richard had reveled in the wonder of seeing the world with such clarity, we saw Dr. Klein. The news was not good: "The tumor is back."

Richard's eyes followed her pencil as she traced the paintball-like splatters of the tumor in the MRI images of his brain: "Here," near the lobectomy cavity; "here," closer to his frontal lobe, the seat of personality; "and here," between his brain stem and the corpus callosum, where the tumor could finger into his still-healthy left hemisphere.

What makes glioblastoma tumors so difficult to treat is the same thing that makes them fatal: They are shape-shifters, returning again and again in differing forms; that behavior gives rise to their formal name, glioblastoma multiforme. Richard's tumor began as the discrete "marble" removed a year and a half before, then resprouted like multiple mushrooms after a spring rain, necessitating the second surgery; now, it spread tendril-like throughout his entire right brain.

I hadn't considered what the flood of fluid that caused his repeated brain crises implied: new tumor activity. How could I have ignored what was so obvious? Denial. Therapeutic stalling can help us process difficult news, but when denial becomes a habit, it's dangerous, preventing us from acting in a crisis, whether personal or global.

I shivered. Richard put his arm around me.

"I've sent the scans to Neurosurgery so they can evaluate whether the tumor is operable," Dr. Klein continued. "Honestly, it's so extensive, the chances are slim."

A ghost of a smile crossed Richard's face. "As Dr. Brega said, 'None of your brain is spare.'"

Dr. Klein nodded. Dr. Chen, she reported, thought he might be able to slow the tumor with focused radiation treatments, but he needed to see more detailed scans. "I've put you on the priority list for openings in the MRI calendar." She paused. "It's time to get serious about your end-of-life choices."

Richard nodded. "I don't want extraordinary measures. As for dying, it's not something I look forward to. But I want to die at home in hospice care, and Suz is okay with that."

I leaned in to kiss him, wordless in the face of this new reality: Richard's end. He and Dr. Klein switched to discussing potential clinical trials. Richard was interested in those using DNA from the patient's tumor to make a custom vaccine against the cancer cells. One was at UC San Francisco, the other at Duke University. Dr. Klein said the VA would be supportive of either.

"Miracles happen," she added. "I've seen some."

Richard was focused and clear, his left brain on the job; I was trapped in a blur of emotions. We were Mars and Venus. That's the nature of grief: No two of us, no matter how close, go through that process of coming to terms with endings in the same way, on the same timetable. There is no one correct path. Ours was parting.

We stopped at Dad's on the way home. I recounted the news as I filled his fridge.

"Let me know how I can help," he said. I hugged him, touched by his support but too numb to respond.

Later, as I drove the winding route into the mountains, I reminded Richard to call Molly.

"I can help research clinical trials, Dad," I heard her say. "What are you looking for?"

At home that night, I called my brother. "Think about what you need to strengthen the circle around you," he said.

I couldn't think. I couldn't even cry. I knew that I would be fine

—eventually; I just needed time, as Dad had said when Mom was failing. Richard had decided it was okay to die at home. That was his prerogative. I hadn't decided it was okay for him to die at all.

The morning after that starry night at Lucia Lodge, we walked hand in hand from our cabin to the lodge for breakfast. In the dining room, with its wainscoting of local redwood, we sat at one of the charmingly mismatched antique tables and tucked into an assortment of fruit, yogurt, eggs, and pastries. I opened the road atlas. We had planned to follow the coast south as far as Santa Barbara, but we were both tired. It was day sixteen, and we had already driven 2,700 miles. Home was at least another 1,200 miles away, depending on our route.

"I think we should turn inland, toward home," Richard said, as he munched a Danish. "Let's head east to Bakersfield and then go over Tehachapi Pass. If we go north up Owens Valley, we can wave at Mount Whitney and then catch Highway 50 and follow it to Salida."

I grinned. His right brain could no longer decipher the map, but his left brain still remembered the geography we had explored together over the years.

"It's been a wonderful trip," he added, "especially being here at Lucia." He paused, face regretful. "It's a long way home—I wish I could help drive."

I did, too. I wished I didn't have to shoulder his care alone, plus serve as driver and guide. . .. For a moment, I let myself feel my exhaustion. Tears threatened. I couldn't cry now. So I squared my shoulders, lifted my chin, and lied without a qualm. "I'm fine. Your company is all I need."

On Friday after the Monday morning when we learned that Richard's tumor had roared back, we drove to Denver for the MRI Dr. Chen had requested. Richard had evaluated clinical trials and decided to apply to the one at UCSF, since Molly lived nearby. "The three of us could explore the city and its outdoor art."

In a photo on my desk, Richard and Molly stand arm in arm, grinning at the camera. Her dark hair blows in the spring wind; his reading glasses are perched atop the shaved dome of his head. Next to them is a boulder bisected by a jagged crack, part of *Drawn Stone*, an Andy Goldsworthy sculpture at the de Young Museum, newly rebuilt after the Loma Prieta earthquake. Goldsworthy's piece alludes to quake-created fractures in what seems like solid ground. It was spring 2008, and we were visiting Molly in San Francisco for the first time. A few hours after I shot the picture, we argued bitterly with her, fracturing the bonds of our relationship. We were still mending that rift when her daddy saw birds and was diagnosed with brain cancer. She was thirty-two when he died—a split that cracked both our hearts.

The morning after the MRI, Richard and I resolved to take our time and make the most of what we had—to *live* his life, end and all. To start, we lingered at a favorite coffee shop in a spacious repurposed industrial building on the banks of the Platte River.

I sipped hot chocolate and journaled; Richard drank dark-roast coffee and called Molly to chat. We ambled along the river and watched kayakers and ducks bob in the current. On the road home, Richard spotted a band of bighorn sheep ewes munching spring-green grass near the highway. We stopped and rolled down the car windows to inhale the fragrances of moist earth and life awakening. I thought about the irony: Outside was spring, and in our lives together, fall was ceding to winter.

Three days later, we were back in Denver to talk with Dr. Chen. The focused radiation treatments, he said, could slow the tumor but would not stop it. "There's not much time—about a month. After that, the tumor will be too large, radiation too dangerous." He continued, "Apply to the trial; if you don't get in, call me. We will start as quickly as we can."

*A month.* The drumbeat of time quickened.

Richard and I held hands as we left. I asked if he wanted to visit *Corpus Callosum.*

"Not this time. Let's go to the VA and get copies of my records for the clinical trial."

"Okay," I said. "I love you."

"That makes me a lucky guy." He spun me in a circle and kissed me, his arms strong, joy infectious. I laughed, almost forgetting the clock ticking on the tumor, and on our life together.

Richard snoozed as I drove across the city, woke for the obligatory stop at Dad's, and snoozed again while I drove home over the mountains. I woke him when I backed the car into the garage. He was slow; I was exhausted. He carried his briefcase into the house and then plopped down in his chair in the living room. I unpacked the car, put away the food, emptied our duffel, and sorted the accumulated mail while Richard sat, silent, staring into space.

"Are you okay?" I finally asked.

"I'm just resting." His voice was slow.

"Can you help?"

"Not really."

My right arm hurled the tangelo I had just picked up before I even felt the blast of anger. The fruit hit the refrigerator door and splattered, spraying a wide arc of juice and pulp.

"Fuck! I can't do this all myself!" I shouted. "I can't do it all myself!"

"What's wrong?" Richard asked, voice flat.

"I'm exhausted from driving you to Denver and back twice in a week. You say you can't help, but you assume I'll always help you. That's what's wrong!" I stomped outside, slamming the door behind me, and paced the back porch. I could feel Richard slipping away. I was angry at the tumor, angry at fate, angry at the cancer that had hijacked my healthy husband and sent us into this death spiral.

And I was scared. To my bones. I needed Richard, and I was losing him. I began to shiver. I went back inside.

Richard was on his hands and knees, trying to clean the kitchen floor, and had succeeded only in smearing sticky tangelo pulp across the bamboo-plank surface.

"I'm doing my best." He looked up, face miserable.

"I know, my sweetie." I knelt and wrapped my arms around him. "I know. I'm sorry." I picked up the chunks of pulp and wiped the floor and the fridge door.

He held out his hand. "Let's go to bed."

I put mine in his. "Okay."

I helped Richard through brushing his teeth and changing into pajamas. We both fell asleep right away; I woke not long after that, heart racing. I tried yoga breathing. I tried calming thoughts.

I got up and paced the dark house. Nothing helped. Finally, desperate, I woke Richard. "Can I snuggle on your shoulder?"

He cuddled me sleepily. "What's wrong?"

I smothered hysterical laughter. What was *not* wrong? I tried to explain and burst into tears. I couldn't stop crying. I got up for tissues and collapsed on the toilet seat in the bathroom, sobbing. Richard came in, groggy, and laid his hands atop my head. I leaned into his legs and continued to sob. "I'm losing you! I'm losing you."

"I'm here now. Come back to bed with me. I can be comforting."

I did. Richard fell asleep again. I lay awake, alone.

The next morning, Richard pulled me close. I laid my head on his shoulder. "Are you still mad?" he asked.

"No, I think I know what was happening: I was letting go of the illusion of control. I can't cure your brain cancer. I can't save you. The only thing I can do is let go of that attempt to control so that I can do my best to love and appreciate you in whatever time we have together."

I raised my head. Tears slid down Richard's cheeks.

"I'm sorry," I said. My voice broke. "I wish I had that magic wand."

"Neither of us does. I'm moved by your ability to see. Thank you. I love you so."

Control is an illusion. That may be the most important lesson of death, whether the death of someone we love, of civility and democracy, or of the earth as we know it. No matter how skilled and compassionate we are, we can no more control the course of life than we can steer a hurricane. Nor can—or *should*—we "control" our emotions, whether grief or anger or joy. We can only bring our best self, whatever that means, to each moment and each day.

I dried his tears and mine with the sleeve of my nightshirt. We snuggled. He stroked my breasts. "Want to make love?" he asked.

"With you?"

It was an old joke. Richard laughed, as I'd hoped he would.

We kissed and caressed until we were both aroused. Only Richard's penis, always so reliable, didn't cooperate: The tip bent to one side, floppy. He slipped inside me awkwardly. We moved together, but nothing happened. I stroked his face and willed myself not to cry. I kissed him. "Love is about more than lovemaking."

Richard smiled, yawned, and rolled over. "I think I'll doze some more."

He was asleep in moments. I blew my nose, wiped away tears, and unrolled my yoga mat beside the bed, timing my breath with his. We were together still. That had to be enough. A line from a poem by our friend, poet Rosemerry Wahtola Trommer, came into my mind: "So much to ripen, if given the chance." And oh, I wanted that chance!

I'd like to say that in that moment I embraced the obvious truth: We wouldn't grow old together. There would be no retirement years; no time for Richard to explore his notebook full of sculpture ideas, for road trips, for seeing new birds; no slow walks into the sunset of our days. I didn't. Instead, I clung to the fact that we still had each other, ignoring the fact that the tumor fingering through Richard's right brain had irrevocably changed him, and thus our "we." His ripening was reaching its peak; mine, perhaps, was still to come.

Richard began to sleep more. His left hand sometimes went numb; he struggled to button his shirts. I began helping him dress and undress. I tried to stay cheerful; he tried to be patient. We were both pretending. It was the best we could do.

On a Friday toward the end of April, the call came from the clinical director of the UCSF trial. I watched my love's face fall at the news: He did not qualify for admission.

"Would you mind talking to my wife?" Richard said after a minute. "I'm still pretty sharp intellectually, but I get confused sometimes." He handed me the phone. The director explained that Richard's tumor was too extensive.

I swallowed despair and asked what he would recommend.

"Start on Avastin infusions right away to cut off the tumor's blood supply."

I gulped. Avastin—the deadly drug of last resort, with side effects including strokes and fatal internal bleeding. "Thank you. We'll consider it."

"I'm sorry we can't admit him. Please call if you have questions. Good luck."

Dad and my Norwegian cousin Halvard visited that weekend. Richard enjoyed the company, beaming even when he napped. They left Sunday evening; on Monday, we woke to spring rain drumming on our roof. Richard carefully built a fire in the woodstove while I made breakfast. Later, I wrote in my journal as Richard looked at *Boundaries*, by the sculptor Maya Lin, creator of the Vietnam War Memorial.

"Do you think the Avastin route makes sense?" he asked suddenly.

I took a breath and picked my words carefully. "I do. Before, it seemed too dangerous. Now"—I paused, searching for encouragement, not just for him but for both of us—"it's a way to buy time." I reached for Richard's hand.

He nodded. "I'm coming to accept that."

Acceptance shifts as conditions shift. For us, at that moment, it meant accepting Avastin as our last hope. And accepting the end that "last" implied—an end to us.


Later, we walked the creek path in a misty drizzle. Richard spotted a bird perched among the ivory blossoms of a sand-cherry tree.

He squinted. "Is that a hermit thrush?"

I wiped water from my glasses. "Looks like it."

He whistled a hermit thrush's fluting call. The bird fluted a few notes in response.

Richard's smile bloomed. "I love that sound."


As we were getting ready for bed that night, Richard's left side collapsed. He slid to the floor in slow motion. I rushed over and helped him up.

"I'm okay." Even his voice was slow. "I don't know what happened. I was walking; then my hand went numb. Then I wasn't walking."

"Left side, right brain." I spoke before thinking and watched Richard's face as the implication dawned: the tumor. "I'm going to call Fran in Neurosurgery tomorrow and see if they can get you in. I'll ask if we can see Dr. Klein, too, to talk about Avastin. Okay?"

"I guess it's time," he said, his voice sad.

Acceptance takes courage—the strength born of love.

*tumor growing*
*you sing to hermit thrush*
*thrush sings back*

# chapter twenty

Day Sixteen

## Odometer Reading: 2,778 Miles

After breakfast, I packed the car and we set off, first following the coast to Cambria and then cutting inland. As the highway climbed steep ridges, lush coastal scrub changed to brittle grassland and scattered oak trees. The temperature rose, too, as we exchanged the moderating ocean for inland heat. We stopped at the crest to scan one last time for the huge silhouettes of California condors. None appeared. An American kestrel hovered nearby, pointed wings beating against the wind, tail fanning like a rudder as the bird hunted for grasshoppers.

Later, we stopped for lunch at a weedy pullout in the dappled shade of spreading oaks. The car thermometer read ninety-five degrees—too hot. But Richard needed to pee and I needed food. He ducked behind a fat oak trunk. A California scrub-jay scolded him in its scratchy voice, azure back shimmering. Richard chuckled at the jay while I set up our camp chairs and prepared our simple picnic.

I opened the road atlas as I munched baby carrots. "Shall we explore the Carrizo Plain," I asked, "or aim straight for the desert?"

"Desert," he said, chewing an open-faced sandwich of Havarti cheese on crusty sourdough bread. "I've been missing Joshua trees and roadrunners."

"Okay."

In the car, his eyes closed as we sped east toward the Mojave Desert and then, a thousand or so miles down the road, home.

That spring, we began a different kind of turning for home: going "home" in the spiritual sense of approaching the end of Richard's life in a mindful way. The day after his collapse in the bathroom, we met with Dr. Brega. The tumor was indeed too large to remove, she said. "You'd lose too much of your right brain."

Then we saw Dr. Klein, who suggested steroids to resolve his left-side issues. Richard looked at me.

I swallowed. "If they'll help, I'm all for it, crankiness or no."

We discussed Avastin. "It isn't a cure," Dr. Klein said, honest as always. "But I think it would give you better quality of life in the time you have—which we hope is long. There's a small chance you could have a stroke, lose your ability to function—to talk, walk, be the 'you' we know now."

"How small?" Richard asked.

"Statistically, about one in a thousand."

He nodded. Tears ran down my face.

"Don't start! Or I'll be crying, too," she said with mock fierceness as she handed me the tissues.

Richard looked at me again.

"Okay," I managed, voice choking.

Dr. Klein explained the process: Richard would receive an infusion every two weeks, assuming his blood pressure and white-blood-cell count stayed in the normal range. That meant coming to Denver twice a month. Dad would like that, I thought—a bright side of sorts.

That evening, Richard asked if I would help him write thank-you cards to his providers at the VA. "I want to let them know while I can that I appreciate what they've done for me."

I wiped my eyes again.

By the next morning, the steroids had already improved his brain function. I had to hustle to keep up with his brisk strides as we distributed the cards.

It was April 27, and I wondered how long we had.

Acceptance is a bumpy process, like grief. Some days we are able to face what is ahead, some not.

A week later, we snuggled in bed at dawn, watching sunrise tint the peaks rose pink. "What are you thinking?" I asked.

"My biggest mental challenge is the need to hold open two opposing possibilities for the future. While we have to be prepared for the worst outcome, for the possibility that the rapidly growing tumor in my right brain will end my life in weeks or months—"

"Hold that thought." I dashed to the bathroom for a tissue, tears flowing. Richard's logical left brain was as brilliant and dominant as ever; I was awash in a flood tide of emotions. Mars and Venus. Tissues in hand, I returned to bed. "Sorry. Go ahead."

"At the same time, we can't abandon the hope that the Avastin infusions will help my immune system stop the tumor."

Taking dexamethasone greatly improved Richard's brain function: He could again button his shirts, build a fire in our woodstove, and help in other ways. But it couldn't repair the damage the tumor had already wreaked. His short-term memory and ability to sequence tasks were gone—every morning, we made a list of what he wanted to do that day and then checked it at mealtimes. Some days he struggled just to type an email, locating letters on the keyboard one by one. Other days he enjoyed reading, but he no longer picked up his notebook to write or sketch. And the dex rekindled the hair-trigger temper. I wasn't sure if Richard noticed. I didn't ask, wary of provoking his anger.

As we snuggled that morning, Richard continued, "I remember a resident at the hospital talking about dissecting a cadaver brain and how much she learned from the experience. I'd like to donate my body to the medical school; I like the idea of continuing to teach, of my death offering a learning experience for someone."

I swallowed tears. "I'll find out how to set that up."

Tears leaked from his eyes, too. "Physical parting will be hard," he said.

"We'll never really part, my sweetie. You've shaped who I am, and I've shaped you, too."

Richard was doing his best to live with an increasingly impaired right brain, and with the knowledge that his life span was short. I was doing my best to meet his needs, hold our household together, live out our time with love, and prepare to let him go. We were simply doing our best to live, period. Breath by breath, step by step, day by day. Sometimes that's the most we can do, and if we do it with love, that's pretty damn good.

As he slowly washed the dishes after lunch that day, he said, tone curiously detached, "I feel as if I'm being forced to leave you —as if at gunpoint."

I wrapped my arms around him from behind and inhaled his patchouli-soap fragrance. "Even when we're not together"—I cleared my throat—"you'll always be in my heart."

"Thank you," he said calmly, and continued carefully wiping a plate.

After stacking the dishes on the counter, Richard headed to the bedroom for a nap. I stowed the dishes so I could find them again. He now put the dishes "away" in random locations—in the freezer, for instance, or atop the barbecue on the back porch. Then I gathered my garden tools and headed outside to begin spring-tidying in our mountain-prairie yard. I needed plant time to steady me.

The front yard prairie was my first restoration project on our formerly industrial property. While Richard designed the house, I researched the natural history of our bare and weedy ground, poring over historic photos and records from the 1880s, when Salida's streets were first platted. Back then, our place was windswept shortgrass prairie. I hoped to coax that native grassland to return and help heal our long-neglected site.

The bunchgrass and wildflower seeds I scattered in an experimental plot the first fall sprouted abundantly the next spring— much to my delight and to the astonishment of our supplier of native-plant seeds. It felt as if the blighted soil had simply been waiting. Those pioneering plants in turn "called in" a whole web of insects, microbes, birds, and animals, from shimmering hummingbirds and graceful butterflies to big-jawed harvester ants, the "earthworms" that enrich our high-desert soil. A project that began as an experiment grew into a flourishing natural community. And unlike a lawn, it needed little water, no chemicals, and no mowing, only an annual trim that mimicked the spring grazing of native pronghorn.

As I snipped and raked dead foliage and flower stalks, I inhaled the rich fragrance of soil organisms waking up and uncovered the tender green of plant life renewing itself—and renewing me, kneeling on the warm ground, an acolyte to that mysterious and quotidian process.

Near one of the rounded granite boulders Richard had placed in the yard as natural sculptures, I uncovered the first wildflowers: starry pink blossoms crowning a softball-size cactus. I fetched Richard from his nap. He knelt beside me to admire the cactus flowers, his smile glowing. In that moment, hope sang louder than grief.

A week later, we returned to Denver for Richard's first Avastin infusion, bringing a box with my young tomato, eggplant, and basil plants for Dr. Klein. As we walked through the halls of the hospital, the greenery elicited smiles from passersby. We found seats in the crowded atrium, and Richard placed the box of plants between his legs.

"Tomato!"

I looked up at the sound of a hoarse voice. A vet whom I had seen many times but never heard speak stopped his electric wheelchair next to Richard. Richard lifted the box. The man slowly extended one hand, fingers trembling, to caress the fragrant leaves.

A smile creased his face. "Tomato!" he croaked again. Then he punched the chair's controls and lurched on, still smiling.

Plants are our breathing buddies, and so much more. Their green presence exudes wordless comfort: Surgical patients placed in rooms with live plants report less pain, anxiety, stress, and fatigue than patients in rooms lacking plants. Plants boost our health and happiness—they root us right back into the earth, our home.

I looked at the clinic doorway. Dr. Klein waved, and we walked over to meet her.

Richard handed her the box. "For you."

"All of them?" She beamed. "They're so big!"

Later, Richard led the way upstairs to the infusion center and walked confidently right past the turn. I pointed to the sign. He laughed. "At least I'm close."

The infusion nurse showed us to a room furnished with reclining chairs, each with a companion IV pump and side chair. Richard settled into a recliner. The nurse set up his IV and attached a bag of saline for hydration, after which came dexamethasone, ondansetron (for nausea), and finally Avastin. I sat beside him and wrote while the pump hummed, the drugs dripped into his veins, and visitors stopped by. Natalie checked in, Char from Oncology delivered Dr. Klein's thanks, Kathi from Pharmacy reviewed Richard's prescriptions, and Sarah from Palliative Care brought the forms for body donation.

Three hours later, we were on the road home. Richard dozed while I drove, relieved at how easy the first infusion had been.

Recovery was not so easy. Richard's mood turned dark, and he quit talking. I gave him two days, stretching my patience. On the third morning, I set a plate of freshly baked chocolate-chip cookies next to his coffee. "Do you think you're depressed?" I asked, tone neutral.

"I'm gravely ill, and there's misery all around."

Sun streamed into the living room. The spicy sweetness of stocks, a bouquet sent by a friend, mingled with the cookie aroma. I heard a house finch warbling in the garden.

"I have a disease of the brain. Experts would say it's grave," Richard said with exaggerated patience, the way he would lecture a particularly dense lawyer in cross-examination. "Therefore, I'm gravely ill and life is miserable."

I lost it. I smacked our breakfast bowls into the sink, spoons rattling, and stomped outside. I strode around his studio, down the alley, and back again, too mad to appreciate the sky-blue male mountain bluebird—the first of the year—I startled from its perch. I was over being nice. When I got back to the house, I told Richard I deserved better and so did he.

He lunged at me, face enraged.

I fled outside again. As I paced—frightened now, as well as mad—I remembered Elizabeth Holman's words: "He can't tell he's scaring you." I let out a long breath, walked until I was calm, and then returned to the house.

"I can't fix your brain cancer," I said. "But I can tell you that if you're going to live with it and with me, you need to find a way out of these black moods. They're not fair to either of us."

Richard looked at me, face mutinous, silent.

I soldiered on. "Do you think it would help to meditate? You've said that meditating is your best tool for keeping your emotional balance."

"Maybe," he said, tone grudging. He sipped his coffee and bit into a cookie.

Half an hour and four cookies later, he announced, "I'm going to meditate."

"That sounds good, sweetheart," I said, voice carefully calm.

Meditation did help: Richard's mood improved some. After his second Avastin infusion, though, the darkness seemed worse. I looked up dexamethasone, the cranky drug. When it was taken at high doses like those Richard was getting, the reference said, side effects included depression, aggression, anger, and mania. Great.

Over lunch, I cautiously suggested that we email Dr. Klein about reducing the dose. Richard considered what I said between bites of the chipotle mayo–and–baked salmon sandwich I had made him, and then nodded. I let out a breath.

Dr. Klein responded immediately: "Cut his dose in half." The improvement in Richard's mood was almost as immediate.

After dinner a few days later, we walked to the grocery store hand in hand, enjoying a mild spring evening. Between produce (organic bananas to go with Richard's anticancer cereal) and the freezer section (Cherry Garcia), we ran into our family doctor.

"You look great," Mary said. "When I saw you, I thought, *Could he look any better?*"

Richard grinned. "I tell Suz I hope to be a source of support and joy. For a long time."

I turned away to hide tears, unable to explain the roller coaster of my emotions in a way that Richard's impaired brain could grasp. Another omission, another thing unsaid between us. Another parting.

As we snuggled in bed the next morning, Richard said, "I'm either imagining or feeling greater clarity in my brain, as if things are working more smoothly. It's hard to put into words, and I can't tell if it's some kind of vision or if I really am feeling clearer communication."

"That's wonderful!" I kissed him. I wanted to believe that the good moments would last. I wanted a happy ending, whatever that meant. It's natural to long for a happy ending to any crisis, personal or global, only longing alone won't produce one. It's our actions that matter, and when we act from love, those actions aim truer and are more lasting, propelled by our inner goodness.

Richard's mood was still buoyant two days later when Bill, Lucy, Alice, and Dad arrived for a weekend visit. We met with Dad's lawyer to sort out Dad's affairs, and Richard waded with gusto through legal language that made my eyes cross. Afterward, we walked downtown to eat at a Cambodian restaurant. Richard played host, suggesting food-and-drink pairings, conversing with animation; he even navigated the walk home correctly.

The next morning, he made omelets, flipping and (mostly) catching each, to applause. I cleaned up, feeling cranky. Until I caught myself: He had terminal brain cancer. I didn't.

That evening, Molly arrived and I cooked a feast: blackened salmon drizzled with lime-infused olive oil, Moroccan rice, yams topped with homemade yogurt cheese, and steamed asparagus from the garden. Dessert was Colorado peach halves simmered in red wine with candied ginger and cinnamon, topped by vanilla ice cream. Food as love.

Richard kept everyone laughing through dinner with witty stories, including a hilarious imitation of the stunned expression on the face of the ICU nurse when he had walked in unaided.

Molly stayed on for "Dad time" after everyone else left. She and Richard walked to the river, talked over coffee, and sat on the front porch, watching hummingbirds zip among the wildflowers. After she left, Richard napped through the next few days, still smiling.

*wings trilling*
*hummingbird flashes feathers*
*bright as your smile*

## chapter twenty-one

## Day Sixteen

### Odometer Reading: 2,880 Miles

From the hillside under the spreading oaks where we ate our picnic lunch, we descended into California's Central Valley, once a shimmering expanse of waterfowl-filled marshes scribed by meandering streams. Today's valley—drained, laser-leveled, and so drenched in pesticides it's unhealthy for pollinators and people alike—is the poster child for the promise and peril of industrial agriculture. The car thermometer read ninety-nine degrees. Richard dozed while I drove, foot on the accelerator, air conditioner blasting, mourning the lost richness of the valley and its native inhabitants, creators of spectacular pictograph panels whose stories we can no longer read.

That spring and summer of Avastin, I struggled to find time for normality within the infusion schedule. Every two weeks, we hit the road for Denver for two days: one day with Dad; the next, an appointment with Dr. Klein, followed by the three-hour infusion.

Back at home, we took several days to recover, which left us little more than a week before we had to set out for the next infusion. We crammed as much living into those interludes as possible: walks to the post office and the river, and meals with friends. We watched funny movies—I introduced Richard to kids' animated films, and he laughed his way through *Shrek* and *Finding Nemo*—and we sat in our sunny living room, reading and writing, just being together.

After Richard's fourth infusion, in mid-June, I drove us to Arkansas to visit his family. As we crossed western Oklahoma on the first evening, the car thermometer read 105 degrees at sunset. Along the roadside, I spotted clusters of tenpetal blazingstar, a wildflower that unfurls palm-size, ivory flowers at twilight an invitation to hovering moths. I stopped and set up our camp chairs near a clump in bud. Richard's smile bloomed as the starry flowers opened.

At his sister's house the next night, Richard woke around midnight and headed to the bathroom, footsteps echoing on the wood hall floor. A few minutes later, feeling a vague uneasiness, I got up to check on him. He was circling the bedroom across the hall in the dark, half-naked.

"Where is the toilet?" His whisper was both cranky and frantic. "I can't find the toilet."

I steered him into the bathroom. When he returned to bed, I asked what had happened.

"I couldn't find the toilet in the dark."

"Oh, sweetie! I'm sorry." I reminded him of his promise to Dr. Klein that he would turn on a light to orient himself at night in strange places.

"This isn't a strange place," he said, impatient. "And I didn't want to wake you."

I took a breath and chose honesty: "Now I'm wide awake and my heart is racing because I found you wandering—penis out—in the wrong room. That behavior could have tragic consequences."

"Of what sort?" Richard's voice was testy.

"The police shoot you when you walk outside, naked and confused."

I could feel the gears of his intellect turning before he spoke.

"Confusion happens. I need to recognize and plan for it. I resolve to stop when I'm confused, take a few breaths, and center myself."

If only it were so easy! I bit off hysterical laughter. His left brain was formidable, but it couldn't grasp the subtleties of behavior the damaged right could no longer convey. Nor could I explain in a way that would reach him. "That's a good idea, sweetie," I said, letting go.

We snuggled; he fell asleep. I lay awake, as I often did, this time thinking about compassion and Richard's impaired right brain. I couldn't save him. I could only do my best to practice compassion and love for him as he was now, for all the now we had.

Letting go with compassion and grace is one of life's most difficult lessons, and one of the most necessary, in a world where change—like it or not—is constant.

A few days later, crossing eastern Colorado's vast plains on the way to Denver for Richard's next infusion, I spotted a sign for Sand Creek Massacre National Historic Site, a place we had long wanted to visit to honor its horrific history. In November 1864, Army colonel John Chivington and his company attacked an Arapaho and Cheyenne camp there, despite peace flags flying from the tepee poles. At least two hundred Indians died, mostly women and children.

I paused and then turned down the gravel road while Richard slept. A few miles later, he woke as we descended a low hill, aiming toward a line of cottonwood trees marking the creek and massacre site. We walked slowly through the prairie, his steps hesitant, his balance disturbed by the noise of the rushing wind. We stopped to admire lemon-yellow flowers on sprawling prickly pear cactus, and the new green leaves of buffalo grass. He smiled at the silvery fluting of a distant meadowlark, followed by a different song: a burst of wheezy and burbly notes close by. That singer, a large sparrow with bright chestnut and black head markings, hopped along the track a few yards away. "Lark sparrow!" I said.

Richard nodded, his face radiant with awe. The sparrow sang again. We listened and then turned and walked at Richard's halting pace to the car.

Richard tipped his seat back and closed his eyes. "Thank you. I'm going to rest now."

Halfway back to the highway, I spotted a domed object about the size of a ball cap in the center of the gravel road. I stopped. "It's a box turtle."

Richard opened his eyes and rolled down his window. I got out of the car, prairie wind whipping my hair. The turtle withdrew into his shell (vivid red eyes gave away his sex). I admired the markings and reached down to carry the turtle to safety. As I hefted the surprisingly solid creature, a stream of pee issued from the shell, just missing my feet.

Richard laughed. "I have that problem, too, Turtle," he said. The turtle's head peeked out. Richard waved a greeting. I set the turtle gently in the prairie and drove on.

*ponderous in domed shell*
*turtle inches across road*
*then whoosh! safe*

The next morning, Dr. Klein had good news from Richard's MRIs: The glioblastoma appeared less active. "Do you want to continue with the Avastin?" she asked him. "I'd like to keep you on it indefinitely if it's not impairing your quality of life too much."

"Yes." Richard spoke without hesitation.

Dr. Klein looked at me. "Are you okay with that?"

Tears filled my eyes. Continuing the Avastin meant the rest of our days would be governed by the infusion schedule. I swallowed the lump in my throat. "If it's what Richard wants, yes."

At home that night I lay awake, troubled. I wanted to support Richard's choices, but I was no longer sure his tumor-damaged brain could fully evaluate them. Avastin was, in Dr. Klein's blunt words, "poison." Were we doing the right thing? What did "impairing his quality of life" mean? It wasn't clear. The truth is, there is no single correct answer; what is right will vary with the person, their culture and family, and their health. Any answer will change as those variables change. That's true of most important life questions, whether about how we live and die or how to respond to racism and the other toxic "isms" that divide us. We must trust our gut, listen well, act with love and compassion, and reevaluate as life unfolds.

Richard woke. "Rest your head on my shoulder. Tell me what's wrong."

"It's that word 'indefinitely,'" I said, sidestepping the more complex issues. "The infusions are a reminder that our time together is finite. I guess I'm grieving."

Richard was quiet. Then he began reciting the Ralph Waldo Emerson quote that hung on our bedroom wall, a circle of calligraphy within a round frame he had made years before with scraps of teak from a furniture project. "Our life is an apprenticeship to the truth . . ."

I joined in, our voices twining, his steady, mine teary: "that around every circle another can be drawn. That there is no end in nature, but every end is a beginning."

Biology and experience had taught me the truth of Emerson's words: Life as a whole continues, even as our individual forms do not. Our physical selves eventually decay, disarticulating into the building blocks of atoms and molecules, which are inevitably rearranged into new forms, whether single-celled microbes, hummingbirds, the flowers that feed them, turtles, or humans.

That natural recycling shapes my spiritual beliefs. To me, the sacredness innate in this universe comes not from God or gods; it springs from life's continual reinvention, the spark that ignites inanimate matter into respiring beings over and over in the circle where the end is also a beginning. Before, I understood Emerson's words in the abstract. Now, their truth was personal.

"A circle has an endpoint," Richard said. "We have to realize that I am approaching mine."

I searched for comforting words. "Your circle will live on in Molly and your work, and in the people you have inspired throughout your life."

"Thank you," he said, voice drowsy. We snuggled and drifted off to sleep.

I woke later to Richard's legs twitching; he had kicked off our Pendleton blanket. I smoothed it over him, remembering the day I bought it, after my solo backpack trip in Wyoming.

After six days alone and ninety-plus miles of hiking, I left the wilderness sure of one thing: I loved Richard and Molly, and somehow, we would make our new family work. I didn't have a plan, but I trusted my heart. Browsing in a store in Jackson, I spotted a pile of brightly colored Pendleton blankets. I unfolded one, admiring the midnight-blue background with colorful geometric bands in a traditional Native American design. Stroking its soft nap, I heard the voices of a group of Crow Indian ladies in my Cody neighbor, Terry's, kitchen. They were chattering as they beaded, telling raucous and sometimes risqué stories in Crow, and translating them with much laughter into English for my benefit. Terry unfolded a Pendleton blanket she had just bought as a gift. Rose Plenty Good set down the moccasins she was beading to stroke the brushed-wool surface. "Skinny Pale Girl [their teasing name for me], do you know the pattern?" I shook my head, and she took my freckled hand in her wrinkled one and traced the peak-shaped triangles ("where the spirits live"), topped by mounds of rain clouds ("life") and bands of rainbows ("beauty").

I heard Rose's voice in my memory as I admired that same design on the Pendleton blanket in the store in Jackson. It was the perfect gift for Richard and Molly. Then I checked the price tag and gulped. Still, I could see the blanket on our bed—the bed we didn't have yet—as a vivid symbol of the love we had found and the home we would make.

Tucked under that blanket again, Richard quieted. I lay awake, tears trickling down my face. *How long? What will I do when he's gone? I don't know. All I know is us, now.*

That Saturday was our annual Cabefest bash and the celebration of Richard's sixty-first birthday. I was determined that we would fete his continuing existence with what he called "an attitude of celebration and gratitude." Midmorning, Richard carried our red paisley yard umbrellas out to the boule court and opened them, signaling party time. Molly helped me move the steel trestle table Richard had designed and built for gallery shows out to the front porch to hold platters of food: quiche baked by Dave at Plough-boy, the local-food market he and Kerry ran; three kinds of muffins; a melon-and-strawberry salad; and homemade yogurt. We poured ice over bottles of champagne and beer in a galvanized tub.

As guests began to arrive, Richard stood on the front walk, beaming and accepting hugs. The yard filled with friends and family eating, talking, and laughing. Molly got her daddy to break out the boule; teams formed and play began. Bystanders sipped mimosas in the shade, cheering or good-naturedly heckling each point. If Richard's once-precise pitches were wobbly and his measuring eye slow, no matter—the joy on his face was contagious. I stayed busy tending the party, distracting myself from wondering if this was his last Cabefest.

Before infusion number six, we headed to Carpenter Ranch to work on our project. When I parked under the big spruce tree that shaded the bunkhouse, Richard woke, alert and helpful. He carried bags and boxes inside without being asked, opened the windows to let in the breeze, and patiently shooed out mosquitoes. (I would have squashed them; Richard's inner Buddhist didn't allow the needless taking of any lives, even bloodsucking ones.)

At sunset, we stood arm in arm on the porch and watched golden light illuminate the Yampa River Canyon in the distance. A sandhill crane bugled from a nearby river meadow.

Richard grinned. "I'm a lucky guy."

We both slept soundly that night.

The next morning, we worked with a landscape architect to "ground-truth"—lay out and adjust our plan. Later, Richard napped while I helped the Nature Conservancy interns and their crew leader collect limestone boulders to use in the new garden. After lunch, Richard demonstrated how to use the rocks to sculpt linear "outcrops," evoking the cliff strata they had come from. When he headed inside for another nap, one of the interns commented, "He's cool. You'd never know he had a brain tumor. His hands know what to do with rocks."

I repeated the comment to Richard later. He grinned again. "That's good to hear. Maybe when we get home, I'll feel like working on a sculpture."

After dinner the next day, we sat on the deck overlooking the garden-to-be. When I recounted a funny story from the day's filming of a video on pollinators, Richard tipped his head back and laughed from deep in his belly. His smile lit his whole face. I reached for his hand and listened to swallows chatter overhead and the throaty calls of distant sandhill cranes.

Richard's smile was one of his greatest charms. His normal expression was thoughtful, but when he smiled—whether sweet and joyful or tinged with mischief—it was like the sun shone on the whole world.

In a photo snapped during our backyard wedding reception nearly three decades earlier, Richard leaned against the wall of the greenhouse, his hand on my shoulder. I sat with four-year-old Molly in my lap, her dark cap of hair shining, cheeks rounded in a smile that echoed her daddy's. I was grinning, dimples creased. Richard positively beamed, his whole being illuminated.

Two days after we took that photo, we shoehorned the three of us into our Subaru hatchback, packed with everything it could hold, and drove to West Virginia and Richard's first teaching post. Richard would try to fit in but would resign ten months later; Molly would be heartbreakingly ill; I would be homesick for the West's wide skies and the fragrance of sagebrush. In the picture, though, those struggles were the unknown future. We were happy in that moment.

In the moment at Carpenter, what lay ahead were the most difficult months of our lives. But right then, Richard was smiling and I was relaxed, not worrying or grieving. The feel of his hand in mine, the sound of a tractor engine puttering, the birdcalls, the smell of sagebrush on the breeze, and the sunset painting the sky were enough.

Endings can be painful and unspeakably grim. But there are

also times of joy, contentment, and love. Times that carry us out of the darkness and into the light of simply being.

"How are things going?" Dr. Klein asked in Denver two days later.

Richard responded by asking if he could go off the steroids. "I don't like knowing my moods scare Susan."

"Yes," she said. "If you both stay alert for the symptoms of brain swelling. Tell me *immediately* if you notice anything."

At home the next day, Richard woke in a lighthearted mood. He laughed when I told a silly joke and delighted me by joking back. He spotted the first blossom on the miniature water lily in the water garden in a pot I had placed outside our bedroom door and came to find me to share the surprise. Like the flower, his smile bloomed. He was carefree, more like the old Richard, before the brain surgeries and dexamethasone. He seemed much less . . .

"Fretful," he suggested when I attempted to articulate the difference. "I feel more like me."

"That's a wonderful gift," I said.

*There could be more good days*, I thought. *Maybe many, many more.*

*water lily bud*
*sprout from mud and darkness—*
*magenta surprise*

# chapter twenty-two

*Day Seventeen*

Odometer Reading: 2,999 Miles

A s the air conditioner in our motel room in Ridgecrest, California, rattled in rhythm with Richard's snores, I lay awake, brain still buzzing, reliving the day's drive, including the moment descending Tehachapi Pass when Richard spotted the first punkrocker forms of Joshua trees in the dusk. "Hello, Joshua trees!"

He loved their sculptural shapes, the Dr. Seuss–ian "arms" spiked with needle-tipped leaves. I loved their bond with tiny, dusk-colored moths. In late spring, Joshua trees sprout spikes of ivory flowers that shimmer in the moonlight, attracting those moths. Females pollinate the flowers and then drill a hole in each flower's ovary and lay an egg. The growing moth larva eats some —but not all—of the developing seeds. Without the moth's pollination, Joshua trees cannot reproduce; without those seeds, no moth larvae survive. They need each other—like we do.

After Richard went off dexamethasone, his good mood persisted and he began talking about sculptures he wanted to work on.

Only talk was all he did.

"It's his vision," Elizabeth Holman said when I asked why he was stuck. "His brain sees in only two dimensions now, so he literally can't envision how to start. If you can get him going, his hands will likely remember what to do."

I knew just the project. For Mother's Day the previous year, Richard had given me three tons of local red flagstone, along with a promise to use it to lay a sculptural patio in the dirt courtyard off our bedroom. Then came brain surgery number two, my mother's decline, and the new tumor activity. The slabs of rock were still stacked in the dirt outside our bedroom door.

The last Sunday of July, Richard sipped coffee in the living room, a sudoku puzzle open. "If I gather tools," I asked, "would you help me lay the first stone for the patio?"

"I don't think I have the energy." He looked sad.

"You can sit nearby and direct me," I said. "I'll prepare the ground; you pick a stone and show me how to set it."

"I can try." His voice sounded doubtful.

"That'll work," I said, cheerfully determined.

He settled into a chair by the sliding glass door while I hacked at the hard ground, pried out rocks, and then screened sand to use as a bed for the flagstones. Sweat formed a line down my back. My muscles sang. When the ground looked ready, I asked Richard to check it. He laid his level on the newly smooth surface, squinted at the bubble, and pronounced it good. Then he eyed the stacked slabs and selected one measuring about two by three feet, weighing, he guessed, about 250 pounds.

"How on earth are we going to move it?" I asked.

Richard grinned. "Watch." He tilted the flagstone onto one edge and eased a long scrap of wood underneath, and then carefully slid the heavy stone on this "sled" to the prepared area. On a count of three, we lifted the flagstone, grunting, and lowered it into place. It rocked slightly. Richard tilted the slab back on its edge; I releveled the bed; we replaced the stone—success!

Elizabeth was right. Once he had his hands on the rock, his muscles remembered what to do.

It was two o'clock by the time we had laid two more flagstones. I sent Richard inside, still smiling, to wash up and rest. I cleaned and stowed tools, then prepared sandwiches with yogurt cheese, salmon, and fresh dill and woke him to eat a late lunch.

Richard paused, sandwich in hand. "I've been thinking about that patio for months, and feeling bad. I just couldn't see the project all the way through, so I was reluctant to start. Once you got me going, I knew just what to do. That feels good. Thank you."

I knuckled tears from my eyes. "Thank you for teaching me. I love you."

The next weekend, we laid half a dozen more flagstones in the same way—I preparing the ground, Richard selecting the flags. By the time we quit, I was sore and sweaty—and proud of myself for learning a new skill. Richard was simply happy to work with rocks again. "Collaborating feels good," he said, as we got ready for bed that night.

I looked out at the patio in progress and smiled. "We do good work."

As always, he drifted off to sleep right away and I lay awake, remembering the other time I had talked him into letting me help on a project.

It was October, several years before the birds. Richard was in the midst of replacing the leaking metal roof of his studio building. He came in for dinner one day, discouraged. He had just finished wrestling the old metal sheets from the decking, and it was taking much longer than he had expected. I reported the weather forecast: ten inches to a foot of snow expected by morning.

"Great," Richard said, voice exhausted. "I've got to get the waterproof membrane on tonight, or that old roof decking will leak like a sieve." The building held his hundreds of tools; his big woodworking machines; his sculpture equipment, his books, and his stash of rare wood.

"I can help," I offered, as I served up dinner. Richard looked at me doubtfully, seeing, I am sure, my lack of muscles and construction experience. "I'm serious," I said. "Anyone can lay out waterproofing membrane. That'll free you for the skilled stuff: the flashing and brickwork."

He demurred. I pressed—I may be slight, but I am determined. Finally, he gave in.

After dinner, I followed him across the alley and climbed the ladder to the steeply pitched roof. Richard showed me how to unroll the black membrane over the wood planks (shiny side up, sticky side down) and how to steady the heavy, ten-foot-wide rolls so their weight wouldn't pull me off the steep roof. I began work: squat, unroll a length, make sure it overlapped the row below, straighten the roll, duck-walk to unroll more, stand to stretch back and thigh muscles, squat again, repeat.

At first, Richard hovered. After a few minutes, I apparently passed the test, because he went back to fashioning metal flashings for the chimneys and stabilizing the brick parapets. We worked in companionable silence as evening slid into night. When it was too dark to see, he climbed down the ladder to fetch his portable lights. I stretched and scanned the sky.

Uh-oh. Clouds blotted out the stars to the southwest, the direction our storms come from. I shivered but said nothing. Richard hooked up the lights; we got back to work.

Around midnight, the wind picked up, and we scrambled to secure loose edges. Suddenly, rain splattered out of the darkness. The upper quarter of the decking was still bare, exposed. Richard raced down the ladder and returned with two huge blue tarps. I spread them out, and as they rippled in the wind, he nailed the edges. *Thwack! Thwack! Thwack!*

Ten minutes later, the rain stopped as abruptly as it had begun. I tugged on his arm.

"The rain has quit. We can finish!" We listened to the night: no patter of rain.

He removed the tarps, and I recommenced rolling out membrane.

Just before 2:00 a.m., I laid the last row of waterproofing; Richard replaced the ridge cap. The roof was tight. We staggered down the ladder with armfuls of tools, then walked arm in arm to the house and fell into bed, exhausted and aching.

By midmorning the next day, eight inches of snow blanketed the ground, with more falling. We slogged over to check the studio—no leaks.

That night didn't change our roles: Richard continued being tool guy and master of all construction projects, and I continued running our household and garden. What did change was my self-confidence: I learned that I was physically and mentally stronger than I had realized. I would need every bit of that belief in my ability to tackle almost anything to dig myself out of the financial and emotional hole his death left me in.

His self-confidence bolstered by the patio work, Richard began taking his morning coffee outside to survey his rock yard, the boulders and industrial materials he had collected for future sculptures. I used the time to journal and catch up on household tasks. Life felt good again. Richard could no longer bake sculptural loaves of bread, drive, or even type an email, but his mood was sunny. And he was thinking sculpture.

One morning, he came into my office and held out his hand. "I've picked out the rocks for the Mayer water feature. Want to see?" We walked outside, and he pointed to a roughly cube-shaped rock about eighteen inches on each side; on one face, thin, sparkling layers of mica traced a V shape reminiscent of Richard's arms upraised in joy.

That rock was the base, he explained, where the clients' Buddha statue would sit. Water would trickle down a flagstone slab rising behind the statue, echoing the shape of the Flatirons, a distinctive rock formation visible in the distance from their garden. As he described it, I struggled to stem tears. I could envision the work; I could see him creating it. What I couldn't see was whether the tumor would allow him the time.

That evening, Richard brought up the Big Trip, our postponed Pacific Coast expedition. "I can't drive, but I can help with the organizing. And I think I'm still good company."

"You are excellent company." That hadn't always been true, but it was right then. I leaned over to kiss him. "Let's do it."

Richard talked happily about visiting Bill and Lucy and the girls, eating fresh seafood and drinking local beer, seeing Molly in San Francisco, and spending time in Big Sur.

All of which we had now done. We were headed home, on the final leg of our road trip and our time. After leaving Ridgefield, we drove north, climbing the dark basalt flow that separates the Owens Valley from the low desert, leaving behind Joshua trees and their waving limbs. The glacier-sculpted granite peaks of the Sierra Nevadas rose on the east in a formidable wall.

We ate our picnic lunch in the shade of cottonwood trees along a rushing creek at Big Pine, remembering the time we climbed nearby Mount Whitney, the peak the Shoshone call *Tumanguya*. It was the autumn after West Virginia, and we had parted with Molly at her mom's and then hit the road, searching the West for a place to make a home for the three of us. One hot October night, we camped under date palms in Death Valley, the lowest point on the North American continent, at 282 feet below sea level, and impulsively decided to climb Mount Whitney, 14,505 feet, the highest point in the continental United States. Twenty-four hours later, we parked at the Whitney Portal trailhead, a twenty-two-mile and steeply uphill round-trip hike from the summit.

We rose before dawn the next day and set off in waning starlight. By midmorning, we had climbed above the tree line and could see the switchbacks leading to the knife-edged ridge below the summit. Noon found us puffing our way step by step in the thin air to the peak itself. We stood hand in hand, taking in the view to the east over waves of desert ranges to Death Valley in the hazy distance, and to the west over the glacier-carved lakes and ridges where my mother had hiked in the '30s and '40s with my granddad Milner and where my family had backpacked when I was a kid. Then Richard and I plopped down, backs against a sun-warmed boulder, and ate our way through lunch: salami, cheese, crackers and peanut butter, Death Valley dates, oranges, and a chocolate bar.

"I'm going to rest my eyes," Richard said, as he savored the last bite.

My storm sense tingled. "Not now." I tugged him to his feet. "The weather is changing."

By the time we reached the top of the vertiginous switch-backs, gusts swirled around us, hurling icy snowflakes. We hiked steadily downhill in a blizzard and finally reached the trailhead after dark, bone-cold and exhausted.

The next morning, we learned the trail had gotten snowed in and was closed for the winter. We drove north and settled in Olympia in time for Molly to arrive for Christmas.

In mid-August, three weeks after we laid the first flagstones for our new patio, we returned to Denver for Richard's seventh infusion. His left-side blind spot had grown big enough to hide me. And he had lost music: He could no longer whistle birdsongs or even simple tunes.

"It's the tumor, isn't it?" he asked Dr. Klein.

"Let's put you back on the dex," she said, sidestepping his question.

Oblivious, Richard launched happily into describing our plans for the Big Trip.

Dr. Klein looked directly at me. "Leaving sooner is better than later," she said. *Oh.*

She reviewed his bloodwork and approved the infusion, and Richard headed out the door. I waited until he was out of earshot and said, "We should talk about what's ahead."

"We'll make time for that next visit." She hugged me. "Before you leave."

I blew my nose and dashed after Richard, who missed the turn again.

At home, he resumed his daily routine: morning coffee and sudoku, reading, thinking about sculpture, and visiting with friends. After lunch, he napped, meditated, and skied on his Nor-dicTrack. On weekends, we laid more flagstones for the patio. His mood remained sunny.

At the end of August, I threw a dinner party to celebrate that Richard was, in his words, "still here." He cheerfully set the table in his own brain-impaired fashion (spoons on the left, forks on the right, knives wherever) while I prepared a meal from the garden: fingerling cucumbers and baby carrots with my herbed yo-gurt cheese to start, followed by local eggs poached on a bed of chard and curried rice with sautéed Japanese eggplants. For dessert, we had vanilla gelato topped with strawberries and port. Happy voices filled the house, and I relaxed, listening to Richard's laugh. We could live with brain cancer, I thought, optimistic again.

We returned to Denver for Richard's eighth infusion the first of September. He reported to Dr. Klein with pride that his brain was working much better—which was at least partly true, although his balance and left-side issues were worse—and that the dex didn't seem to be causing black moods, which was entirely true and a great relief to both of us.

"Can we talk about what to expect as the tumor gets worse?" I asked.

Dr. Klein looked at Richard. "Is that okay?"

"Absolutely," he said. "I imagine I'll just wake up one morning without a pulse."

"That would be convenient," she replied, voice dry. "What is most likely is a gradual decline." His brain function would slowly diminish, she said. "You've seen some of that already with memory and spatial issues." (He had gotten confused that morning walking inside from the parking garage.) Then would come physical decline and, she said, "Eventually, you'll succumb."

Dr. Klein's eyes glistened with tears. I reached for Richard's hand. He squeezed mine.

"I want to refer you to hospice," she said. "It's early, but that way you'll have a chance to get to know them, and they to know you, before it's more difficult."

"Can we wait until after the Big Trip?" I asked. Richard nodded his agreement.

"Of course." She hugged us, and we headed upstairs to the infusion center. Richard walked right past the familiar door and laughed when I tugged his arm. "It's a good thing I have you to keep me out of trouble."

As I aimed him into the center, I hoped fervently that I could.


On the drive home, Richard slept, my hand in his. Near the top of Kenosha Pass, I looked idly at a pond where we often spotted ducks. Something large, furry, and brown moved on the opposite shore. I slowed and pulled off the highway. Richard woke, and I handed him the binoculars. A young male moose, antlers covered in lush velvet, knelt on gangly legs at the water's edge, gobbling mouthfuls of grass.

"Wow!" Richard breathed, once his brain and the lenses aligned. "I'm a lucky guy."

*grazing in muck*
*coat rich chocolate, rack velvet—*
*ecstatic moose*

That night in bed, I said, "It was two years ago yesterday that you saw birds."

He pulled me close. "We've learned a lot on this journey that neither of us would have asked for."

"We've done our best to take it with love and thoughtfulness . . ." My voice broke.

"To honor the 'body of love' between us," he added.

"It feels like we're as ready as we can be for whatever's ahead," I said, battling tears.

What was ahead scared the hell out of me, but I was determined not to let Richard see that. My resolve was to honor his journey as best I could.

The "care" in "caregiving" comes first, no matter how difficult.

Richard woke three times during the night to pee. He apologized the next morning.

"It's a side effect of the dex, sweetie," I said. "There's not a lot we can do about it."

That evening, voice serious as he sat on the toilet, he said, "I'm having a conversation with my urethral sphincter and my bladder."

"Oh." I kept my voice carefully neutral. "What are you saying?"

"I'm relaying my expectations about them performing in a way that I can go all night without getting up to pee, so I won't disturb you."

"Thank you." I was immensely touched by his intention. But I could see a flaw in his usually sound logic. I suggested that he express his appreciation for his bladder and urethral sphincter first, and then ask if they could help him wake as few times as possible. "That way, you're enlisting their cooperation. You need them to let you know if you do have to go."

"You're right," he said. "I want them to alert me. I like the idea of appreciating them."

The next morning, perched on the toilet again, he said, "I'm appreciating my urethral sphincter and bladder."

"Good," I struggled not to let a chuckle escape.

"I'm thanking them for helping me not get up to pee more than once."

"Good," I repeated, thinking, *Could this journey be any more surreal?*

Silly question. It would be, and soon.

*brain circuits blocked*
*Richard talks with his body —*
*word to cell and synapse*

chapter  twenty-three

*Day Eighteen*

Odometer Reading: 3,493 Miles

Richard stopped in front of the wall-size relief map inside the visitor center at Great Basin National Park. "Show me where we've been."

I traced our journey over the past two and a half weeks, from home in South-Central Colorado to Carpenter Ranch, and then through Wyoming's southwestern corner to Lava Hot Springs in Idaho. My finger slid across the Snake River Plains, crossed the mighty Snake River on the border with Oregon, and then moved north to Pendleton. West along the Columbia River to Portland, and north again to Olympia for our weekend of Tweits.

Richard's eyes followed my finger south to the mouth of the Columbia River, and then meandering with the curving coast through Oregon and California to San Francisco and that weekend with Molly. Then Monterey, the Big Sur coast, and that magical night at Lucia Lodge. From there, my finger headed southeast on our route to Ridgecrest in the Mojave Desert and, the next day, north along the Sierras, and the long drive across Nevada's desert basins and skinny mountain ranges to Great Basin National Park.

Last, I traced that day's route east on US 50 toward Moab and home.

"We've come a long way," he said, face sad. "It's time to go home."

Home meant hospice care. The end of our larger journey.

The day before, Richard woke as the car crested a narrow mountain range in central Nevada. He looked at the rounded boulders on either side of the highway and said, "This looks like where we found the hawk."

The year before his bird hallucinations, we were headed in the opposite direction across Nevada, Richard at the wheel, to visit Molly in San Francisco. Topping a rocky summit on a lonely stretch of road, Richard spotted a wing flapping on the ground— a hawk, downed.

"Go back!" I cried. He whipped a U-turn. A female red-tailed hawk lay on her chest next to the pavement, head raised in alarm, fierce golden-brown eyes turned toward us. One wing flopped, broken. Her body was immobile, except for her head.

"Her back must be broken," Richard said. "There's nothing we can do."

"No!" Tears choked my voice. "We can move her farther from the roadside at least."

He shrugged and dug out an old army blanket, and we walked toward the bird. The hawk hissed, not yielding. Mindful of her sharp beak, Richard carefully wrapped the blanket around her broken body and carried the bundle down the hill through a scattering of rabbitbrush and sagebrush.

"Let's put her in the shade," I said.

He laid the hawk gently on the dry earth under a sagebrush, then carefully unwrapped the blanket. The hawk stared at us, eyes unblinking. "Oh, honey," I said, choking back more tears, "I'm so sorry. But at least here you've got shade and quiet. You can die in peace."

I bowed to the hawk, out of respect for her life, and then reached for Richard's hand. We walked back to the car, shook out and refolded the blanket, and drove on.

I wiped tears from my eyes at the memory. "I think we found the hawk farther west."

"I'm glad we moved her downhill so she could die in peace."

"Me too," I said. I didn't add the thought that rose unbidden. We were headed home to do just that for Richard: give him a place to die in peace.

Our sincere and probably naive intention was to live well and embrace his ending. Practicing that intention was, of course, neither simple nor easy.

Our second night at home after the Big Trip, I woke at midnight when Richard turned on his flashlight and headed to the bathroom. He returned to bed and was asleep a few minutes later; sleep eluded me.

I got up and padded through the dark house to the kitchen. I looked out the window at the night sky. The view of the stars and the infinite vastness of space, usually comforting, now seemed simply bleak. That afternoon, Richard's hospice nurse, Will, whose dark hair and quirky smile reminded me of a younger Richard, and Nathan, the hospice social worker, had come by for their initial visit. Richard greeted them and invited them to tour his studio and see his sculpture work—as if theirs was a social call, not an acknowledgment of his impending death.

*Does he not notice how his hands shake and his steps falter? How much he sleeps? Is he being strong for me?* I couldn't tell.

I curled up on the living room couch, wrapped in a throw, and listened to Richard's snores from the bedroom. Before brain cancer, I thought, on a wave of self-pity, he would have come looking for me, folded me in his arms, and said, "Tell me what's wrong. We'll figure it out together." That Richard was lost to the tumor born of his own cells and now growing unchecked in his right brain. Those cells and their genetic error would kill him.

Tears trickled from my eyes and turned to a flood, pouring down my face. I rocked back and forth, sobbing, arms wrapped around my chest for comfort. I tried to calm myself, but the sobs grew into a wail that wouldn't hush, a keening from deep within, as if my very cells were grieving. I keened and rocked, keened and rocked until I was spent, then dragged myself to our bathroom to wash my face and blow my nose.

"Where were you?" Richard's voice was slow, groggy. "I woke and you weren't here."

"In the living room," I said, my throat as raw as I felt. "I didn't want to disturb you."

"I was confused; I thought there was a baby crying," he said. "Come to bed and rest your head on my shoulder. Tell me what's wrong."

I tamped down hysterical laughter. He was dying. What wasn't wrong? "It's everything, sweetie. I'm exhausted and overwhelmed and afraid."

He snuggled close. "I'm afraid, too. But we have each other."

I took a deep breath, anger flooding me. We didn't have each other anymore! It was all on me. The wave ebbed as quickly as it had come. It wasn't his fault that he couldn't grasp the changes. Although we were still physically together, I was keenly aware that our parting had already begun. His strong fingers massaged my neck, something he had once done every night, before the cancer stole his energy and awareness.

"I'm letting go, I guess," I finally said.

Richard was quiet for a moment. "The most important thing hasn't changed."

"What's that?"

"That body of love. Love can do wonders. I don't have much energy right now." He cleared his throat. "But I'm determined to approach each day with celebration and gratitude. I'm still here with you, and I'm grateful for that."

He drifted off to sleep, fingers lax on my neck. I lay awake, my head pillowed on his shoulder. The year before, Richard had written in my birthday card, *With this birthday, we mark the time when half of your life up to now has been spent with me. Thank you for the great gift of your company.*

Those decades together were coming to an end. I was approaching a solo life, something I had never imagined. I always assumed—we both did—that I would die first. It was a reasonable assumption, given my chronic illness and Richard's lifelong robust health. Only life doesn't abide by assumptions. They are merely a comforting illusion; we are not in charge. Fiction, I thought as I drifted off to sleep, is easier. You can write happy endings, believable or not.

The next morning, Richard selected a chocolate out of the hospice comfort basket Will and Nathan had left. He unwrapped it, popped the sweet into his mouth, and then carefully smoothed and read the words inside the foil wrapper. "Oh," he said.

I looked up. His eyes were full of tears. "What?"

He passed me the wrapper with its message: *Love every moment.* I wiped my eyes and reached for his hand. "That could be our motto."

He nodded. "It's how we've been living."

I saved that wrapper, tucked under the lid of the porcelain jar holding Richard's ashes.

Our fourth morning at home, we were practicing yoga when Richard's left side suddenly collapsed. I helped him up, relieved he wasn't hurt, and suggested as calmly as I could that he sit and meditate next to me. The guy who was once, well, arrogant about his strength agreed without argument. Another letting-go.

That night he stopped, toothbrush and toothpaste in hand, confused.

"You put the toothpaste on the brush," I said, and turned away to hide tears.

"Right." He chuckled. "I knew that once."

Two weeks after returning home from the Big Trip, we woke to fresh snow. I made a fire in the woodstove, gave Richard his morning drugs, and wrote them on his chart. When he had eaten breakfast and was comfortably ensconced with his coffee and dark chocolate, I readied the guest cottage for Grant Pound, who was due in for a weekend of sculpture apprenticeship. Then I washed three loads of laundry and walked to the post office. Richard napped and talked with Molly on the phone.

That night, he missed the toilet entirely and peed on the floor. I didn't discover the yellow puddle until the next morning.

"I can feel my sculpture self awakening," Richard said, as he climbed the two steps from the studio to the house after Grant's visit, leaning on the cane he now used for balance. That afternoon, he announced he would join me to walk to the post office, a first since we had gotten home from the Big Trip. He set off with confidence, beaming with delight. After two blocks, though, his steps began to falter. I turned him around, pointed to our house, and said, "Go straight home, take your meds, and rest."

Richard smiled, leaned in for a kiss, and crossed the street, steps wobbling. I watched him go and then headed on. Ten minutes later, my phone buzzed.

"I'm standing in front of Safeway." Richard's voice was weak. "I thought I was supposed to wait for you so we could buy flowers."

"Oh, sweetie!" I said. "You must be exhausted. You were going home—remember?"

"Go get him!" Toni, our silversmith friend, hissed in my ear. "You're scaring me!"

I shook my head and said into the phone, "Walk straight home now, sweetie." I hung up and said to Toni, "He's okay. This is our life now."

As we got ready for bed that night, I asked Richard what had happened.

"I got confused. I wanted to get you flowers. You're working so hard to take care of me."

My heart broke. The brilliant economics professor and expert witness, the sculptor who could discuss art and Buddhism with equal insight, was no longer safe on his own.

Richard picked up his toothbrush. "Brain cancer sucks."

"Yup." I wrapped my arms around him.

He squinted and carefully squeezed toothpaste onto the brush. "I still consider myself a fortunate guy. I have your love and companionship."

"You always will. Even when we're no longer together physically, you'll have my love."

"And you'll have mine," he said, and then began carefully brushing his teeth.

Dr. Klein called that Friday to check in. When I reported that Richard's spirits were good but he was weakening rapidly, she asked if we were still planning to drive to Arkansas to visit his family.

"We are," I said.

"Go now," she responded. "I don't want you stuck there if his condition deteriorates."

*Oh.* I took a deep breath. Leaving that day meant driving until midnight in order to reach his sister, Tish's, house the next day. *But if that's what we need to do*, I thought, mentally squaring my shoulders, *I'll do it.* "Okay. I'll call Richard's hospice nurse."

"Good idea—now, let me talk to Richard." I handed the phone to Richard and called Will.

Will agreed: "Don't wait. I'll alert the hospice organization there in case you need them."

Two hours later, we turned onto Highway 50 and my heart

lifted simply to be back on the road. Afternoon light glowed through gold cottonwood leaves; snow-dusted peaks glistened in the distance. Richard dozed. I sang along with Emmylou Harris and "Take That Ride."

An hour and a half from home, he woke. "I have to pee."

I pulled off the road, raced around the car, and opened his door—too late. *Damn it!* I helped him change and then got out his dinner, an egg-and-potato burrito with the green chile sauce safely tucked inside. I fashioned a bib of paper towels, just in case.

"I lost track of time. I'm sorry," I said, as I pulled back onto the highway. "No wonder you couldn't hold it."

He chuckled through a mouthful of burrito. "That makes me feel better. At least we know my bladder's good for more than an hour." In a few weeks, he would "graduate" to adult diapers, a passage neither of us imagined then.

Later, the full moon rose, pale yellow and round, over dark mesas. I woke Richard and pointed.

"That's the moon we share." His voice was slow. He smiled and drifted back to sleep.

Tears streamed down my face. Our lives were racing toward his ending, as if time's accelerator were stuck on full bore.

We had planned to spend several days at Tish's house. But within twenty-four hours, Richard lay prone on her couch, eyes shut, strength gone. Watching him, I said quietly to Tish, "He's fading. I think we should head home tomorrow. I'm sorry." She shook her head, eyes sad.

When we left the next morning, Tish hugged Richard. "Thank you for coming to visit," she said. Her face said, *Goodbye.*

Three hours later, west of Tulsa, Oklahoma, I spotted a hundred or so American white pelicans in migration, soaring high overhead on long wings. The sun glinted off white plumage and ink-black wingtips as the big birds spiraled upward. I pulled over, woke Richard, and opened the sunroof so he could see the birds while reclining.

"Wow!" he breathed. We watched the gyre until the pelicans reached a layer of southward-flowing air and coasted, wide wings extended, out of sight.

Richard reached for my hand. "Thank you." He closed his eyes. I drove on.

Twenty minutes later, he announced, "I have to pee."

I looked ahead and saw only waving prairie and scattered cows. I pulled over to the side, opened his door, and helped him out. He was plainly visible to passing traffic, but I no longer cared. He was dying; the usual rules didn't apply.

By the time we reached Colorado the next day, Richard could barely walk. He lay in the passenger seat, slowly eating lunch. "I'm sorry I'm so exhausted." Even his voice was frail.

I took my hand off the steering wheel to cover his and gathered both words and courage. "It seems to me you're in the phase of life where we have to let go of a lot." He nodded, still chewing. "This is hard to say, but it's important. . .." I cleared tears clogging my throat. "I want you to know you can take your time letting go. You don't need my permission, either."

He squeezed my hand. "What a beautiful benediction."

I blinked away fresh tears. "I don't want to part. But I don't have any choice." I gulped. "Our love will last when we don't."

"It will." Richard's eyes glistened. He took another bite of his sandwich.

*autumn wind buffets car—*
*my hands clench the wheel*
*my heart lets go*

Forty-five minutes later, he began to squirm. I pulled off by a farm field and helped him out. He was leaning against the car, peeing, when my phone buzzed. It was Will, asking where we were. "Two hours away," I responded.

"Good. I've been worried," he said.

A smile flitted across Richard's puffy face. "Me too."

Will heard Richard's halting voice. "I'll meet you when you get home."

Will arrived as I finished unloading the car. Richard lay on our bed, propped on pillows.

"I came straight inside to pee," Richard said, "and then collapsed on the bathroom floor." I stared, shocked. He hadn't told me. "I sort of folded slowly," he said. "I didn't hurt myself."

"I think it's time for you to use a walker," Will said. "And a commode chair at night."

I looked at Richard's mutinous face. "I'm going to take cover," I said, making it a joke.

Will's mouth twitched. "That's why I took a step back out of the line of fire."

Richard shut his eyes: "Hospice equipment. Apparently, letting go requires new tools."

Will's mobile eyebrows flew upward. He snorted.

I laughed and kissed Richard. "I'm glad your sense of humor is still intact."

# chapter twenty-four

## Day Nineteen

### Odometer Reading: 3,822 Miles

The morning of day nineteen, we lingered in a coffeehouse in Moab, Utah, in no hurry to hit the road for home. It was midday and hot by the time we set out. Just outside town, we stopped to explore a new pedestrian bridge arching over the Colorado River's muscular flow.

As Richard got out of the car, I asked, "Do you want your hat?"

"I don't think I need to worry about dying of skin cancer," he said, his tone dry.

My eyes watered. "Good point." Road trip rule number eight: no needless worrying.

While Richard examined the design of the arching steel bridge, I scanned the wide ribbon of riparian forest along the river. Those riverside plants and the relationships they nurture are vital to the health of both the waterway and the surrounding desert. For decades, this riparian thread had been sick, the diverse native forest choked out by a toxic monoculture of invasive Eurasian salt cedars. Now though, something had changed: I realized with excitement that the salt cedars were dead, their gray skeletons buried in new growth of willows and gangly cottonwood trees already alive with insects and songbirds. A chat called as swallows swooped over the water; a chrome-hued yellow warbler chased insects in the willows; tiger swallowtail butterflies floated through the new, leafy canopy. I blinked, thrilled.

"Look!" I pointed to the riverbank. "The riparian forest is returning. It's a rebirth, like the phoenix arising from the ashes."

"It's beautiful." Richard's steroid-puffy face shone. "Life returns. That gives me hope."

Me too. Not hope that he would live—we were beyond that. Hope that some beauty would sprout from the ashes of his life's end.

*your death a wildfire*
*reducing "us" to ash*
*will poppies bloom?*

We had been home for almost three weeks when Molly arrived, having taken leave from her job "for the duration." She brought Dad with her from Denver for a weekend visit. At seven thirty the next morning, Bill, Lucy, and Alice appeared at the back door just as I slid muffin pans into the oven. They had driven straight through the night from Washington to spend the weekend. October was passing, Richard was declining, but our family circle held us close.

Bill leaned in for a kiss and sniffed the muffin batter appreciatively. "Good timing."

"You're early." I burrowed into the comfort of his hug.

"We traded off and kept driving. Alice would have driven the whole way if we'd let her."

"And you didn't take advantage of that?" I grinned at sixteen-year-old Alice, as curvy and compact as Lucy. Alice wrinkled her nose the way Mom used to, and grinned back.

The seven of us gathered around Richard's steel-trestle table for breakfast. Richard beamed and slowly, right hand shaking, raised his coffee cup in a toast. "Thank you for coming. I'm a lucky guy."

On Monday, after the Olympia gang left, taking Dad with them, I did yoga in the darkness before dawn. I kept an eye on the eastern horizon, watching for the glimmer of the rising crescent moon. *There!* I woke Richard, helped him into his wheelchair, and rolled him to the patio door just as that bright sliver freed itself from the black horizon.

He squinted at the dark sky. "That's the moon we share."

"And have for a long time," I said.

His hand crept up to grip mine. "We're fortunate."

By eight thirty, I had Richard shaved and bathed, lotioned and dressed. He was sitting at the dining table in his wheelchair, eating breakfast, when Molly came over from the guest apartment. A few minutes later, the first visitors arrived: Kent and Cathy Haruf—he a renowned novelist and one of the kindest, wisest, and most unassuming men I have ever known; she the big-hearted and no-nonsense former hospice volunteer coordinator. Our community circled close, too.

Kent sat down next to Richard and resumed their ongoing

discussion of the meaning of the Buddhist concept of *metta*—lovingkindness—in daily life. Cathy and I retreated to my office to talk. She asked how I was doing. I hedged: "You of all people know that the answer to that question is complicated."

"I'm asking as a friend, not a hospice staffer." She sounded like the schoolteacher she had been, chiding a disappointing student.

"Sorry." Molly joined us as I struggled to articulate my feelings. "He's still so formidable intellectually," I said, "and his spirit is so strong. But he can't tell when he has to pee, or he forgets how to button a shirt and brush his teeth. It's a shock to see the speed of his physical decline. After Mom, I thought I was prepared. Maybe we can't be."

Cathy nodded and turned to Molly.

"It's a shock, as Suz said. But I'm grateful to be here and have the time with him." Tears filled Molly's hazel eyes—her daddy's eyes—and spilled down her cheeks. I fetched tissues.

Cathy hugged us. "You two are shining stars of doing caregiving right."

That night, Richard slept in the hospital bed Will had ordered for him, next to the bed Richard had built for us years before. We slept side by side but no longer skin to skin. More letting go.

Two nights later, I woke abruptly to the noise of Richard attempting to get out of bed.

"Do you need to use the commode?"

"Yes. I was trying to get up without waking you."

I raced around the beds, tripped on the leg of the commode chair, and switched on the light. "Remember, you promised Will you wouldn't get up without help."

"I might have forgotten that," Richard said with a grin.

I kissed him firmly, then helped him to the commode and

back to bed. He fell asleep again; I lay awake, thinking about how to pass on his sculpture concepts. An idea tickled at my mind: Molly, trained in cultural anthropology, could interview her daddy; we could record their conversation and make it available, like the dharma talks he had been listening to, only about his art. Discussing his work would give him a chance to teach again. The more I thought, the more excited I got.

I looked at the clock: five thirty, too early to wake Richard. I got up and slipped down the hall to the dark kitchen. Out the window, orange streetlight glow illuminated snowflakes swirling from low clouds. As I cleaned the woodstove and lit a fire, it occurred to me that Molly, who shared her daddy's love of stone and steel, might like to participate in the sculpting apprenticeship with Grant. And Richard could talk woodworking with his nephew Andrew, who was visiting to spend time with "Unc." I checked the time again: 6:20. I carried a glass of water and Richard's prebreakfast meds to the bedroom and opened the blind. He woke and patted his shoulder. I squeezed onto his narrow bed and spilled out my ideas.

"I've always loved to teach. Talking about my work might be useful."

"And a way of passing on your art practice." With my head pillowed on his shoulder, I felt, rather than saw, his smile.

"You're right. Thank you for the wonderful idea."

I raised my head to smack a playful kiss on his lips. "I thought it was brilliant," I teased.

He chuckled, an echo of his rich laugh. "That's the better word."

After I did yoga, I helped Richard to the commode and then wheeled him into the bathroom for a shave and a sponge bath.

He stood up and leaned against the counter to apply lotion to his skin, now fragile from the steroids. And slowly collapsed. I caught him just before he hit the concrete floor. I held him until I could speak without shaking. "Are you okay?"

"Yes, that was scary. Thank you for catching me."

I cleared tears from my throat. "I try," I said lightly, and kissed his head near that sinuous brain-surgery scar. And thought, *I can catch him, but I cannot save him.*

By the time Molly came in the front door an hour later, shaking off snow from her walk across the porch, Richard was sitting at the table in his wheelchair, starting breakfast. I handed her a cup of coffee and explained the art-talk idea. Her eyes lit up. "We could do the first interview right now."

I nodded. "We also thought you might want to join the sculpture sessions with Grant."

"Wow! I definitely want to be in on the studio sessions, Dad. Thank you."

While Richard ate his slow way through breakfast, Molly set her iPad upright to display a photo of his very first basin, *Butterfly-Drinker*, a rough granite river rock with a shallow bowl sculpted in the top. It sat outside on a cedar post in our front-yard meadow, gathering falling snow. "What was your aim with this piece?" Molly asked.

Richard's voice was thready at first but grew stronger as he discussed his work:

"I had the simplest of intentions there, and that was just to introduce a concavity in this very ordinary, completely convex river rock. The consequence was, if you put the rock with the concavity up, it would hold water, and viewers could see 'inside' the rock's rough exterior."

Andrew arrived and pulled up a chair to listen. I poured him a cup of coffee.

"It was an experiment to see if the carving techniques and the idea would work. I made the concavity of a shape and depth I thought would be suitable for butterflies to drink from . . . "

After Richard finished talking, Andrew asked him a question about Craftsman design. CC, a printmaker friend, knocked on the door; Richard sent Andrew to the shop to fetch a book on Craftsman houses, and four heads bent over its pages.

An hour later, Richard began to droop. I shooed everyone but Molly out and wheeled Richard to our bedroom. He drifted off to sleep, still smiling.

The next evening, Molly and I dressed for a girls' night out dinner at our friend Roberta's house. It would be my first night in months away from Richard and caregiving. Grant, Dave, and another artist friend came over to hang out with Richard. At the front door, I stopped, terrified at the idea of leaving him. *What if something happens?* I looked back. Richard sat in his wheelchair at the dining table, a beer in his hand, laughing at something Dave had just said.

"It's okay, Suz." Molly gave me a hug. "Dad needs 'boy time,' too."

I took a deep breath. I knew she was right, but still . . . *This is practice in letting go*, I thought, straightening my shoulders and following Molly into the freezing night. At Roberta's, we were swept inside to warm hugs, glasses of wine, and the rich smells of food cooking.

Over dinner, Roberta clinked her glass for a toast: "Thanks

for taking care of Richard, whom we all love." She handed me a small box. Inside was a bracelet hung with charms each friend had contributed, symbols of my life and work: a flower, a Celtic knot, a fountain-pen nib, a heart-shaped quartz pebble, pearls, a bronze leaf, and a sea turtle—all beaded together with love.

As I circled the table, thanking each woman, Toni the silversmith rushed in, blond braid flying. She thrust a blue silk bag into my hands. "I'm sorry I'm late, but we just finished your gift. It's from me, Jerry, and Susan."

Out poured a stunning necklace: three opals, the largest a tigereye with a sapphire-blue circle in the middle, linked on a gold chain. Ribbonlike twists of gold hung from the middle opal, suspending a miniature pencil that had belonged to my great-grandmother, a California poet and journalist—my foremother in writing. I stared at the necklace, dazzled, near tears.

I swallowed, hugged her, and then raised my glass to the whole group: "You are all gifts—every one of you. Thank you."

Back at home later, Richard dozed in his wheelchair, a smile on his face, clad in only a tailored wool shirt over adult diapers, which he had begun wearing that week. Dave was drying dishes. I surveyed my bare-legged sweetie. "Everything okay?" I asked.

"We had a great evening." Dave's voice was laconic. "There was that moment when we didn't quite make it to the commode on time. We got Richard and the floor cleaned up and continued having fun. His sweatpants are in the laundry basket."

"Thanks for giving him a guys' night." I said.

"No problem."

The charm bracelet jingled on my wrist; the opal necklace hung around my neck. And now, with the thud of pee-sodden sweatpants in the washer, I was back to caregiving. "After the ecstasy, the laundry," as Buddhists say; life itself is the spiritual practice, not those exalted moments when we think we transcend the ordinary.

The next afternoon, I wheeled Richard up the rutted driveway to his studio. "I'm going to have to four-wheel it here," I said. Richard grinned and gripped the wheelchair armrests as I muscled uphill over rocks. Inside the shop, I helped him gather tools and stones for the sculpting session and then listened as Molly and Grant joined him.

"The idea is simply to reverse the curve of the rock's surface and polish the concavity." Richard's voice was slow and thready, but his eyes shone. "To discover the 'window' into the stone. The interplay between the rough native rock and the human intervention—the carving and polishing—reveals the surprise, the inner beauty."

My cell phone buzzed. It was Will. Back to the sacred ordinary I went.

The next day, Molly went out to the studio for sculpting practice while Richard napped. She returned an hour or so later, bearing a river-rounded granite rock about the size and shape of a goose egg. Not quite midway between its ends, a thumb-size indentation sparkled with crystalline reflections, the polished "window" into the rough rock.

"I've got it, Suz! I've got it!" Her wide smile reminded me of her daddy's grin.

Richard woke. I passed him the stone. He cradled it in one

long-fingered hand and rubbed his thumb across the satin-smooth concavity.

"Beautiful." His smile, rare now, bloomed. "You do have it."

That afternoon, Heather and Sienna, our eldest Tweit nieces, arrived for an overnight visit, bringing Heather's youngest, ten-month-old Liam. If they were shocked by Richard's physical decline in the six weeks since we had visited Olympia on the Big Trip, they didn't let on.

We gathered around Richard's table for a dinner made by our baker friends Kathie and Steve: potato-and-green-chile soup, crusty bread, and crisp spinach-and-apple salad. As we ate, we admired Liam and caught up on family news. We didn't talk about death or hospice or brain cancer. For those few hours, life felt blessedly quotidian—an ordinary miracle.

*baby Liam kicks*
*cottonwood leaves rustle*
*your smile still autumn-bright*

# chapter twenty-five

*Day Twenty*

## Odometer Reading: 3,962 Miles

etween Grand Junction and Delta in western Colorado, less than three hours from home, I looked over at Richard. "We can make it home tonight. Or . . ."

"Or we could take our time and look for aspen color somewhere between here and there." He finished my thought, our minds in concert again.

"Exactly."

We discussed heading south to look for aspens around Durango or Pagosa Springs but decided both were too far out of the way. "What about Kebler Pass?" I asked, naming the mountain pass between Paonia and Crested Butte.

"That sounds perfect," Richard said. "We can stay in Delta tonight."

Two days earlier, on the long haul across Nevada, we couldn't wait to get home after two and a half weeks on the road. Now, the closer we got, the less inclined we were to rush.

On the last day of October, Molly sat in a rocking chair next to Richard's hospital bed, reading aloud from the book he had requested: a biography of the Buddha. She read easily until she stumbled over an Indian place name. "This is going to be a problem."

"Because you don't speak Sanskrit—or Pali?" A smile warmed Richard's halting voice.

"There is that."

They laughed, she with his smile and silky, dark hair, his high cheekbones and graceful height; he with the now-steroid-swollen face, the silver stubble around the reverse-question-mark-shaped surgery scar, and his once-muscly body propped up by the hospital bed. *That laughter is the gift of this time,* I thought. Richard and Molly were so alike that sometimes they clashed and pulled back, each hurt and too prideful to reach out. Now, as their time together grew short, they were simply enjoying each other—a blessing, ephemeral and bittersweet.

Richard's decline was accelerating. His physical abilities changed almost daily, the way an infant's do, only in reverse: His firsts were "lasts," not the progress we celebrate on social media. That evening's "last" came when Richard was "too tired" to transfer to the wheelchair for dinner at the dining table. Molly and I brought trays to the bedroom and ate with him there.

Over the next few days, those lasts piled up: I began shaving and sponge-bathing my fastidious love in bed instead of wheeling him to the bathroom. He began wearing his soft night-shirt all day, instead of the crisp button-downs he had favored for as long as I'd known him. Will brought a urinal so I wouldn't have to "dance" Richard's heavy body to the commode so often. One morning, Richard didn't finish his breakfast—another first. That same day, his beautiful smile, always a constant, appeared just once.

My intensely physical man, once so active and adventurous, was now bed-bound, exploring only in his mind in conversations ranging over art theory, the nature of death, lovingkindness, and the merits of local beer. Molly read him books on Buddhist thought; he listened to dharma lectures from his favorite teachers, including Sharon Salzberg, Joan Halifax, and Pema Chödrön. I could feel him leaving us, but I was too exhausted to feel my own emotions. Richard now seemed unruffled, as if he had accepted what was coming. I was present. That was the best I had.

On November 3, I woke just past midnight to Richard's urgent whisper: "Suz! I need to sit on the commode."

I raced around the bed and helped him sit up, lowered his feet to the floor, and pulled his heavy body upright, pirouetting his tall form as if we were dancing, and then lowered him onto the seat, my muscles shaking. He sat, folded over and resting his forehead on the bed, for a long time. Finally, he whispered, "I think I'm done."

I straightened him up, wiped him, and refastened his diapers. Then I lifted and pivoted, waltzing him back to bed. I pulled his legs up and tucked the covers over him.

"Thank you, my sweetie." His eyes slid shut.

I turned to the commode, and my eyes widened. In the bucket floated an enormous bowel movement. I carried the bucket to the bathroom, carefully poured it into the toilet, and flushed. No go. I grabbed the plunger, plunged vigorously, flushed again, plunged again, flushed, plunged, and, finally, success!

I caught a glimpse of myself in the vanity mirror and began giggling. It was nearly one in the morning, and I was standing over the toilet in my night tee and flowered leggings, long hair rumpled, with the plunger held high, like some crazed goddess of plumbing victory. I tried to imagine explaining what was so funny and knew I couldn't. It was hospice humor—you had to have been there. Not that you'd want to be.

As I drifted off to sleep, I remembered Richard's comment when we helped care for his dad: "Wiping your parent's butt is a milestone none of us wants to reach." Wiping my spouse's butt trumped that. *Love every moment*, I reminded myself, with the caveat *as best you can*.

Next thing I knew, it was dawn and Richard needed the urinal.

After dinner on Friday night, I sat next to Richard as he dozed. I listened for Molly, who was in the kitchen. Soon, the rich notes of a flute, the one with the gold head joint she had pleaded for in middle school, floated down the hall. Richard's eyes opened. His head turned toward me, a question on his face.

"That's Molly—she wanted to play for you."

Molly had picked up a flute in grade school and discovered music. Like her daddy, she was so fluent in the language of notes and melody that her playing seemed effortless. Our calendar filled with lessons, recitals, and concerts; our days filled with flute music and arguments about practicing, which she hated to do. After winning a college music scholarship in eighth grade, Molly abruptly quit playing in high school. The more Richard pressed her, the more she resisted.

"She'll play when she's ready," I said. Years passed.

As we listened, Richard smiled for the first time that day. He reached slowly through the bed rails and found my hand, tears glistening in his eyes. "Thank you." After that surprise concert, Molly played every day until he died—and then once more, at the celebration of his life.

On Sunday, our friends Bill and Doris came to help Molly and me with Richard's care before sitting for our regular Buddhist-Quaker silent-worship hour. Once Richard was bathed and shaved, the four of us gathered around his bed. Warm sun poured in through the patio door. As our collective silence spun out, Richard slid into sleep, his breathing even. I struggled to stay awake and be present, aware that our moments were limited. I wanted every single one.

Richard woke as we carried brunch plates and mimosa glasses into the bedroom after worship. He slowly raised his glass. "Thank you for accompanying me on this journey none of us looks forward to . . . but we all take." I wiped my eyes.

A few days later, our friend Marilyn, who was training as a Buddhist hospice chaplain, called to talk to Richard. I handed him the phone and opened my laptop to write—until I heard Richard's voice break. I looked up. Tears slid from his eyes. "I am honored," he said slowly. "Would you like to talk to Susan?" He passed the phone to me, his hand shaking.

I tucked the covers around him and carried the phone to the kitchen.

"He's a bodhisattva," Marilyn said, using the Buddhist word

for an enlightened being. "His spirit just shines through. Thank you for letting me talk with him."

"I'm sure he would want me to thank you," I said, bone-weary, and thought, *He might be an enlightened being, but I still have to wipe his butt.*

"Are you ready?" Marilyn asked, her voice kind.

"Who is?" I countered. I didn't want to talk about it.

She understood. "Thanks for taking care of Richard, from me and all who can't be there to help."

The next day, Grant, Molly, Mark, and Dave conspired to give us "date night," a rare evening alone in a house now always full of hospice staff and visitors. Dave brought soup and bread from the kitchen at Ploughboy; Molly baked an apple crisp. Grant bought roses and fashioned a candle holder from a piston case in Richard's scrap-metal pile.

"We're going out so you can have a quiet, candlelit dinner." Molly bent down to kiss her dad. "We'll call before we come home, just in case."

Richard's face creased into a grin. It took my tired brain a moment to grasp her implication. I started to say something and then shut my mouth. *Let her dream.*

I was in the quiet kitchen, pouring Richard's beer, when he called, "Suz!" I raced to the bedroom for the urinal—too late. I cleaned him up, put on a fresh pull-up, and washed my hands carefully before arranging the dinner tray and carrying it to the bedroom.

We clinked glasses. "I love you."

Richard smiled for the second time that day, a gift. "And I you."

He ate slowly, savoring every bite. I ate mechanically, knowing my body needed the fuel but too weary to truly appreciate it. How many more meals would we share?

"I'm sorry we can't have a real date," he said. "It's been a while since my brain could manage my penis well enough to pee on command, much less make love." He smiled.

I knew exactly when: April 8, seven months before, after we had learned that the tumor had returned this last time. My body remembered the feel of Richard's muscles and his skin, our too-fast rhythm, that urgent wave of release . . . We made love with a kind of hunger that at the time I didn't comprehend, as if it was our last chance. It was. Remembering hurt.

"We had lots of years of wonderful lovemaking, sweetie," I said now. "What matters most now is being together." That wasn't entirely true, but I wanted to believe it. Speaking the truth that I missed our physical connection, missed him already, would only hurt both of us.

He reached for my hand and drifted off to sleep. I opened a novel with a happy ending. I needed to escape into a world where happiness was possible, no matter the ending ahead for us.

*you snore*
*night wind rattles dry leaves*
*I dream happy endings*

At 1:13, I woke abruptly. For one panicked moment, I thought Richard had quit breathing. Then came that urgent whisper: "Suz?"

I leaped out of bed and raced to switch on the light. I positioned the urinal, kneeling on the cold floor. Nothing happened. I felt his diaper. It was soaked. So was the waterproof pad under it, the sheet we used to reposition him, and the fitted sheet under that.

"I'm afraid that horse left the barn already," I said. Richard chuckled.

I carefully rolled his limp form to one side, peeled off the soaked diaper, and cleaned him. Then I bundled the wet sheets and pad on one side of his body and positioned clean sheets and a dry pad on the other side. I turned him onto the clean side, removed the wet layers, and smoothed the dry ones into place. As I pulled the covers over him, I blessed Pam, Mom's hospice nurse, for showing me how to change bedsheets under an incapacitated person, a skill I would never have imagined I would need so soon, and for Richard.

I kissed him, put the disposables in the trash, and tossed the sheets in the washer. It was 2:00 a.m. when I crawled back into bed. I shut my eyes. And heard, "Suz?"

Shit. Indeed—this time it was a bowel movement.


In the morning, Molly asked how date night had gone.

"Suz only had to change me twice." Richard's wavering voice carried wry humor. "She's my official urinal wrangler. And now my diaper wrangler, too."

Molly winced. *That was probably TMI*, I thought, but couldn't suppress my grin at his joke. "That's part of the journey, sweetie," I said. "It was a wonderful date anyway." And didn't add, *Given the circumstances*. That went without saying.

Frost sparkled on the flagstone pavers we had laid just two months before, when Richard woke on Friday and patted his chest with his still-usable right hand, inviting me to snuggle for morning talk time. I clambered over the bed rails and carefully wedged myself alongside his long form. He wrapped his good arm around me.

"I used to say I felt gratitude for being able to walk about on the surface of this extraordinary planet." His voice was halting, just above a whisper. "Now . . ." He paused.

I waited, but no words came. "Now you can't walk. But you can still be grateful to participate in life."

"Yes. That's it. I am."

It was November 11, the end of his sixth week in hospice care. My days were absorbed by feeding, administering medications, changing him, sitting beside him, and soaking up every moment. Staying engaged with the process as Richard rounded the next arc of his life. Everything else was on hold. Afterward, I would begin a new journey, alone. Who that solo me would become, I didn't know, and honestly didn't want to imagine. Sometimes the best we can do is just be present with whatever is happening—hands on, heart open.

Later, Dr. Klein called to check in. I reported that Richard's left side had gone limp.

"He's had two good years," she said, voice sympathetic. "That's almost twice the prognosis for grade-four brain cancer. Most of my patients are not nearly so healthy as he has been."

I calculated. It had actually been two years and eighty-nine days since that August morning when he saw the birds. She was right: He had been relatively healthy, something I supposed I should be grateful for. I wasn't. Yet.

The rest of the day was normal for our lives in hospice care. Friends stopped by; Carol, the volunteer hospice harpist, spent an hour jamming with Molly, strings and flute mingling; Helen, Richard's cheerful hospice aide, gave him a sponge bath and changed his sheets; and Will checked in. By midafternoon, Richard was fretful. I asked if it was time to ration visitors.

"Yes," he said, eyes closed. "Do you mind being gatekeeper?"

"Not at all," I replied. I craved peace and quiet, too.

Love continued to pour in from near and far. Cards bearing sweet and funny messages filled the mailbox, along with books, hand-knitted socks, and a cap "to keep Richard warm," plus gift certificates for local restaurants. Poems arrived via email. A food drive through Ploughboy paid for our groceries. Meals appeared at our front door, plus other offerings: special stones, flower bouquets, and the monthly envelope containing four crisp $100 bills: "For whatever you need."

I was grateful for the support, even as my pride resented our needing help. My emotions were all over the map. One thing was constant: My heart wanted a different ending to our story.

*flowers, socks, and meals*
*your offerings warm our hearts*
*as winter nears*

## chapter twenty-six

## Day Twenty-One

### Odometer Reading: 3,995 Miles

At Moca Joe's Espresso in Delta, Colorado, on the last day of the Big Trip, Richard paused, chocolate-chip muffin in hand, and said, "Thank you for suggesting the Grant apprenticeship. I can see myself getting back to sculpture again."

I smiled. "That's excellent." I slid my hand under the table and knocked quietly on wood. I had no idea what was possible. I knew only that if he was happy, the journey would be easier for all of us.

Later, when we turned off the highway onto the gravel road winding uphill toward Kebler Pass and its miles of aspen groves, Richard reached for my hand. "I love this route," he said, eyes sparkling. "This has been a good trip. Thank you for taking me."

He had already forgotten the bad parts: the times I'd yelled at him because he'd sprayed green chile all over himself, or walked straight into traffic, or whipped out his penis in public; the heat, the dodgy motels, the too-many-miles days. He was remembering the throaty calls of sandhill cranes, eating fresh crab with Bill and Lucy, walking in San Francisco with Molly, the stars at Lucia, seeing new green reclaim the banks of the Colorado River, the love that propelled us. Which, I reminded myself, was what mattered. Always.

Atop the pass, chrome-yellow aspen leaves fluttered around thousands of ivory and olive trunks. I drove slowly, opening the windows to inhale the scent of moist fall earth.

Richard's smile grew. "Coming home to aspen gold is the perfect end to our trip."

It was. Still, I wiped tears from my eyes. "End" was a loaded word in this context.

Seven weeks later, on a Wednesday morning, I lay next to Richard, my head on his shoulder. He reminded me of our conversation on the way home from Arkansas:

"You gave me permission to let go on my own time," he said, voice weak. "I'm doing my best to be aware and mindful, to live out whatever time I have graciously and generously. I want to be a source of support and joy to you."

*Oh God!* He had declined so quickly since that day on Kebler Pass. He was now bed-bound, dependent on me for every aspect of his life, from meals and peeing to simply sitting up. Despite Molly's company and the help of friends and hospice, I felt dreadfully alone and unprepared. I gulped and searched for some wisdom to offer. "Letting go gracefully is an important contribution. You're inspiring us all."

"Like my dad and your mom," he said. "They surprised us by being gracious at the end."

"Exactly. You're inspiring us by being mindful and gracious."

A moment later, he dozed off, his hand slack and warm on my neck, his heartbeat too fast and choppy under my ear. I lay absorbing the feel of his Richard-ness and then got up to begin the day. It was the sixteenth of November. I wondered how much time we had left.

That afternoon, Molly came in from the studio with a basketful of sculpted "comfort rocks" to show her daddy. I had suggested that she carve small river cobbles as gifts for Richard's doctors and primary caregivers. After she and Richard decided on the recipients, Molly spent time sculpting each day. Now, she proudly laid eight rocks on his bed, each the right size to cradle in one hand, with a polished indent that invited stroking.

Richard beamed. "Beautiful work, sweetie." She beamed, too, her smile reflecting his.

He looked at me. "I won't be there to give them the rocks. But you'll do it."

It wasn't a question. My eyes filled. "Of course."

"Thank you." His eyes closed.

I hugged Molly. "Thank you for continuing your daddy's work."

On Monday, November 21—my brother's birthday—Richard woke hungry and asked for his favorite breakfast: a burrito, fruit and yogurt, and superfood juice. I brought him a tray and raised the head of his bed so he could eat. He sipped some juice and then forked up a bite of breakfast burrito and began to chew; I headed back to the kitchen to cook my cereal. As I did, I calculated roughly how many breakfasts I had prepared for Richard over the years—more than ten thousand, I decided. And then I wondered how many times I had taken time to appreciate the simple act of being able to make breakfast for him. Considerably fewer, I guessed. I vowed I would practice from then on.

When I returned, Richard was still chewing. I called my brother to wish him happy birthday. After I hung up, Richard was still chewing. I looked at his tray: He was still working on that first bite. I suggested it was time to swallow.

He shook his head, teeth clicking against each other. I shivered.

Will arrived a few minutes later. I met him at the door and reported Richard's chewing.

"His brain may have forgotten how to swallow," Will said.

*Oh.* Will checked Richard's vitals. His blood pressure was elevated, his pulse fast.

"I think it's time to go to liquid food," Will said. "And to stop all nonessential meds."

Richard nodded, still chewing.

That night, his dinner was his favorite road-trip treat: a pineapple milk shake from Sonic. He sipped half of it and fell asleep. I sat next to him and wrote my weekly "Richard report" to Dr. Klein, Elizabeth Holman, and Natalie. After detailing his physical decline and continued gracious spirit, I paused, and then wrote, "He knows Molly's family leave runs out at the end of this week, after Thanksgiving. I think he's letting go so she can get on with her life." I blew my nose, wiped streaming eyes, and hit "send."

We were beginning his ninth week in hospice care. It would be his last.

I had been married to Richard for almost my entire adult life at that point. Watching his decline, that reminder of our impending parting, I wondered if the fiercely independent woman who had backpacked alone still lived inside me.

That night I dreamed of my child self, perched cross-legged atop a granite boulder in a meadow redolent of pine sap and trail dust: The sun warmed my cap of blond hair. A woodpecker tapped a resonant branch nearby. I looked up from the book in my lap, realized my family was nowhere nearby, took a bite of the cinnamon Pop-Tart in my hand, and continued reading, perfectly content.

I woke in the darkness before dawn in our bedroom, tears leaking from my eyes. I listened for Richard's breaths: slow but regular. I slipped out of bed and padded next door to my office, the dream as real as a memory. I opened my laptop, searched Dad's trip notes from our family travels, and found the meadow.

I was seven years old, Bill nine. We were camping in Grand Teton National Park. Mom planned a day hike to Lake Solitude, high above the tree line and fourteen miles round-trip. We set out early, took a boat across Jenny Lake, and then hiked uphill—very uphill. Six steep and hot miles later, a mile below the lake, I wore out. Mom hiked on, intent on reaching the lake; Dad stayed with Bill and me. I climbed atop a boulder and opened a book from my knapsack.

Later, I looked up and realized Dad and Bill were gone, most likely trailing an interesting bird. Untroubled by being alone in the wild, I read on. Eventually, they reappeared, and then Mom returned. We hiked downhill. Back at the boat dock, Mom put quarters in a pop machine and treated us to cold sodas. I chose root beer.

I closed my laptop and sat listening to Richard's slow breaths.

I could feel the sun on my head, the rough granite pressing against bare skin; I tasted the sarsaparilla in the root beer. I reminded myself that I was still that girl; I could be happy—or at least contented—alone.

The next morning, Tuesday, Richard looked like his old self again. The steroid-induced moon face had vanished overnight, returning the chiseled features of the guy I had fallen in love with exactly a month shy of twenty-nine years before.

Will gestured me into the hall. "I think he's turned the corner."

*Hell!* I remembered Pam gathering us in my folks' living room. One part of me wondered if I was ready to let Richard go. The practical part called Molly to join Will and me in the living room for a family conference that was all too familiar.

"How long do you think he has?" I asked, not entirely sure I wanted to know.

"A day or two at most." Will added, "Of course, Richard does things on his own time."

Molly and I looked at each other and laughed weakly. "He always has."

That night, Molly moved from the bed in the guest cottage to an air mattress on the floor of my office, "just in case."

The next morning, she said, "I want to learn to clean and change Dad." It was November 23, almost two months since we had returned from the Big Trip.

"Okay." We gently turned her daddy onto his side. I showed Molly how to roll up the soiled linens, remove his diaper, clean and change him, and then roll clean linens under his limp form. Molly shouldered the unpleasant work with grace. Richard was sweating and cold by the time we finished. I smoothed the covers and leaned down to kiss him. "I love you, sweetheart."

His eyes opened. He looked from Molly to me. "I love you," he whispered.

At 4:00 a.m. on Thanksgiving, I woke to Richard's urgent "Suz!"

I turned on the light. His jaw was clenched. His body began to spasm; the bicep on his right arm was as hard as rock. I swallowed, feeling sick. "I think it's time for pain meds and muscle relaxants, my sweetie. I know you said that you wanted to stay aware through the process and not use drugs until you needed them. That seems like now. Okay?"

He squeezed my hand, eyes closed.

In the kitchen, I opened the hospice kit, feeling a prickle of déjà vu. I powdered two pills, mixed in a little water, and sucked the slurry into a syringe, just as Pam had taught me. Back in the bedroom, I squirted the syringe into Richard's mouth. And then began the day's medication log—*4:03 a.m.: 1 Haldol, 1 Dilaudid.* By midmorning, after I administered more drugs in consultation with Katie, the weekend hospice nurse, Richard seemed comfortable. I headed out for a walk.

Outside, I strode along, inhaling gulps of cold air and swinging my arms to release the knots in my neck and shoulders. The sky was blue; crows fussed in the trees. The streets seemed oddly quiet until I remembered it was Thanksgiving. *What would I give thanks for?* I wondered. The answer came immediately: *Whatever would ease Richard's passage.*

I shivered, exhausted from being awakened every few hours to change soaked diapers, from the intensity of midwifing the death of a man I loved, from assisting with a journey neither of us had imagined he would travel at age sixty-one—too young.

That night, when Molly and I changed his diaper, it was stained brilliant orange from blood in his urine. Had his kidneys failed? Did it matter? As Will had said, our job was to keep him as comfortable as possible, which to me meant shepherding my partner through this end we hadn't imagined when we'd pledged to live our lives side by side in that long-ago Quaker wedding. I was there to comfort, yes, but also to witness and accompany him on this arc of his path with as much love, wisdom, and compassion as I could muster. And then to continue on without him.

After we finished changing him, Richard's eyes opened.

"Is that Joan?" he whispered, looking toward Molly. She and I looked at each other, her eyes wide.

"No, Dad," she said after a pause. "It's me, Molly."

"I know that." His whisper was impatient. "To your left. Is that Joan sitting next to you on the bed?"

There was no one to Molly's left. At least not that we could see.

My mother thought Richard hung the moon; his intellect and wry sense of humor reminded her of her beloved dad, my grandfather Milner, who died when I was in college. Mom cheered Richard on as if he were her own son. Perhaps, I thought, she had returned to lead him up this final stretch of life's trail. Or perhaps she was a hallucination. We couldn't know. I preferred to believe in Mom's guiding love.

"Mom's feisty and bright spirit has come back to help you," I said, keeping my tone light.

"Yes. You can't see her?" His whisper was puzzled.

"No, sweetie," I said. "Is anyone else here?" I added. Molly stared, tears flowing, eyes huge.

Richard's gaze moved around the room. "No."

"Your granddad Raymond saw family before he died," I told Molly later. "It's a common phenomenon for people near death to see beloved faces." Molly gulped. Her dad was dying. It was all too overwhelming, even without spirit visitors.

Friday was quiet. I got outside twice—a rare treat. Returning from my second walk, I checked the mailbox on the sculptural base Richard had created for my birthday the year before and found a lumpy envelope. I carried it inside and opened it in the bedroom.

"Blanche sent you a beach rock from Washington." I placed the palm-size, wave-smoothed basalt disk under his right hand. Richard's long fingers cupped the flattened rock. I reminded him of the stones on the beach where he and six-year-old Molly had played one summer in Washington. His eyes remained shut; his head moved slightly in a nod.

Molly sat across the room, crocheting a baby blanket for a friend. Her eyes were wet.

"Would you like Geraldine's rock, too?" Another small nod. I found the pebble, part coppery green metamorphic, part speckled granite—a remnant of the wrenching changes that created the valley where we lived—and tucked it into a fold of his T-shirt, over his heart.

"I love you, my sweetheart," I said.

"Love." The whispered word was clear.

Tears closed my throat. Molly swiped her hand across her face. "Love you, Daddy."

> *eyes shut, left hand limp*
> *right hand cradles special rock—*
> *life on the cusp*

Love is waking in the night to wipe the shitty butt and fetch a clean diaper to wrap around bone-thin legs that once rippled with muscle. Love is remembering the beautiful smile while placing the sponge between cracked, dry lips. Love is attention to the rhythm of ragged breathing, kisses on a brow drenched in cold sweat. Love is simply sitting nearby, witnessing, heart as open as it can be. Love is embracing "life's other half," the reality that we all round that circle eventually.

Love is letting go when the time comes, no matter fear and grief, because letting go with love is the best gift we can give in that end that is also a beginning.

# chapter twenty-seven

## Day Twenty-One

### Odometer Reading: 4,154 Miles

After that leisurely drive through the aspens on Kebler Pass, and an equally leisurely and late lunch at a favorite curry restaurant in the mountain town of Crested Butte, we were both suddenly eager to be home. We raced daylight for the final hundred miles of our trip; I backed the car into the garage just as sunset flamed the clouds red and orange.

"Home feels just right," Richard said.

After three weeks on the road, it surely did. The next day, he would begin hospice care. There would be good days and hard days, joyful moments, laughter, and deeply painful ones. We would do our imperfect best to live the ending of his life with love. It was the only way we knew to honor a journey that, as Richard said, we hadn't chosen but we all take.

I woke abruptly at ten past midnight on the Sunday after Thanksgiving and listened: Richard's breaths were fast and shallow. I slid my hand through the bed railings. His right hand twitched rhythmically, beating a weak tattoo on his belly.

"Did you lose Blanche's rock?" I asked. The wheezy breathing paused, his attention palpable. I felt his hand—no basalt disk. I pulled back the covers, found the rock, and tucked it in place. He squeezed my hand slightly, in an echo of his once-strong grip, and curled his fingers around the rock. The other pebble was still tucked in place over his heart.

He burped, his upper body convulsing as his empty stomach clenched. My stomach did, too. I took a steadying breath, knowing instinctively that he could feel my emotions. "It must be time for more meds. I'll be right back."

I tiptoed past my office, where Molly slept soundly. When I returned, Richard unclenched his jaw just enough that I could squirt the drugs into his mouth and slip in a fresh sponge. I slid back under the covers, stuck my hand through the bed rails, and found his hand, still curled around the beach rock. I took a deep breath.

"Remember the Emerson quote?"

As I spoke, I could feel his attention like a focusing of the air between us: "Our life is an apprenticeship to the truth that around every circle another can be drawn. That there is no end in nature, but every end is a beginning."

I swallowed tears. "You're headed for a beginning. I'm going to miss you every day, Molly's going to miss you every day, but our love will be with you. There's love coming to you from all around to buoy you through this passage."

His fingers twitched, squeezing mine.

"It's Sunday. Doris and Bill will come for Meeting, if that's okay."

Another faint squeeze. He burped again, muscles clenching, and then slowly relaxed.

I drifted with the ragged rhythm of Richard's inhales and exhales, not quite sleeping, not entirely awake, as the stars wheeled overhead in the darkness. When dawn light slid around the blinds, I rose stiffly and did yoga, my attention still tuned to his increasingly labored breathing.

An hour later, when Molly woke, I was in the kitchen, making coffee. I hugged her and handed her a cup. "Go sit with your daddy, okay?"

She looked at me, an unspoken question in her eyes. I sniffled. "Not long, I think."

When Doris and Bill arrived, we gathered around Richard's hospital bed. His eyes were closed. His skin had shrunk overnight, molding the bones of his skull like his modeling clay. Doris and Bill greeted Richard and then chatted with Molly. I leaned close and spoke into Richard's ear: "You are closer to that combined ending and beginning, aren't you?"

His right eye slid open, the hazel pupil aimed directly at me. I kissed him gently and closed the lid. "I hate letting you go, but I know it's time. I love you."

Just then, Katie arrived. She warmed her stethoscope, placed it on him, and listened intently, counting his pulse. "I've got a hundred and six."

I turned to see if Molly had noted those data on his chart. When I looked back at Richard, the hair on my neck prickled. His chest had gone still.

"You didn't!" I spoke before thinking. "You didn't just die when I wasn't looking!"

He took a gulp of air. The room was quiet as he breathed.

Once. Twice. Three times. And then stopped. We held our breath. Katie looked at her watch, timing the pause. We knew before she spoke: "He's gone."

Katie hugged Molly and me and then went to the living room to make the official calls. We hugged Richard's still form and then each other, tears flowing. I called my brother, then Dad, then Richard's sister. Then we gathered around Richard and enfolded him in worship one final time.

Afterward, we washed Richard's body, preparing it for the ride to Denver and the university medical school where he would continue teaching. The funeral-home guys knocked on the back door. One was Kevin, a friend from the city public works department. As they transferred Richard's body to the gurney, Kevin said, tone apologetic, "There's no space in our cooler, so he'll have to stay in the coroner's fridge overnight, until the van to Denver fetches him."

I swallowed a bubble of laughter. "I really don't think he'll mind."

They rolled the gurney out the back door. Richard was gone.


Richard had delighted in Sunday brunch at Laughing Ladies, so it seemed natural to close his circle there. I called Kerry and Dave to join us. We convened at the table where Richard had presided in his wheelchair five weeks before during a Tweit-clan visit. We toasted his life with fizzy mimosas, ate eggs Benedict with his favorite green chiles, and told Richard stories through laughter and tears.

As we walked home later, Kerry said, "That was just right. Richard would have loved it."

I swiped at fresh tears at her use of the past tense. He really was gone.

That evening, I sat at the breakfast bar, my ears still tuned toward the now-silent bedroom. Molly joined me. "I want to stay until Tuesday."

"This is your home, sweetie." I swiveled to face her. "Stay as long as you like. Having you here these last five weeks was a gift. Thank you."

We both wiped our eyes.

"I've been thinking about the celebration," I said. "Want to talk about it?" She nodded.

When we had discussed his "after-party," as I called it (he laughed!), Richard's wishes had included food, music, contemplative silence, and time for people to speak if they wished. Molly and I decided to hold the celebration on the Saturday closest to the winter solstice, at Salida's SteamPlant Event Center, next to the sculpture park where Richard's marble-studded *Matriculation* lived.

"It would be great if you feel like playing your flute," I said to Molly.

"I can try," she responded, tearing up.

"That's all we can ever do, sweetie."

She suggested that we provide markers, paper bags, sand, and candles, so that people could create luminarias with messages to Richard on the bags and place them by the sculpture to light his journey. "Wonderful idea!" I added make-your-own luminarias to my list.

After Molly headed back to the guest cottage, I sat on the

couch in the living room next to Richard's empty chair. *Just me, alone now. With no one to tend*, I thought, *I might even sleep all night long. How wonderful would that be?*

Guilt immediately followed. I had no one to tend because the event I had hoped never to experience had come to pass: Richard was dead.

From biology, I understand death as the ultimate recycler, the process of dissolving the physical form of one being into the basic materials used by all of existence. Within minutes after our heartbeat stills, the community of microbes that lives on and in us, fostering our health while we are alive, turns to dissolving that which was us back into atoms and molecules. Once liberated, those building blocks can take new forms. I am comforted by the idea of my body being recycled into new life. For me, what some call heaven would be finding that my components had been incorporated into a big sagebrush plant, rooted in the community and soil of the landscapes I call home. My personal idea of hell is being buried in a decay-resistant casket inside a concrete vault, cut off from that cycle.

I believe that what we call spirit or God is an expression of the ineffable and as-yet-unexplained spark that starts life's pulse in all beings, from bacteria and dandelions to scrub jays and immense blue whales. As I see it, once freed of his body, Richard's spirit soared off to rejoin that life force, what some call the universal consciousness—the sacred impulse that quickens this numinous planet. Thus, both his molecules and his spirit live on, imbuing other lives. Seen this way, death is not an end—it is a passage into life's other half.

I walked out to the front porch. The sky was still luminous, on the cusp between blue and black. And there! The thin silver crescent of the new moon set in the west, as Venus, the planet of love, sparkled nearby.

"That's the moon we share, my love," I spoke aloud, addressing his spirit, which I imagined was still near. "New moon, new beginning."

Venus twinkled, her light refracted by dust in the atmosphere. Earth's shoulder eased toward the planet and that accompanying thin arc of moon. As I watched the two disappear behind the dark horizon, I shivered, shaken again by loss.

I had let Richard go as lovingly as I could. Now, I had to find my own path.

As I slept that night, he breathed beside me in dreams.

I woke to dawn's gray light. Alone.

In a world that echoed with the love we had shared.

*bright evening star*
*Venus rides with tender moon*
*into long night*

# e p i l o g u e

*We are the darkness, as we are, too, the light.*
                                        —Barry Lopez, *Horizon*

Richard and I took one more road trip together. After the packed and emotional celebration of his life, an official letter arrived from the State Anatomical Board at the University of Colorado School of Medicine, acknowledging our donation of Richard's body. He had been placed in "the long program," the letter said; his remains would be returned when it ended. I confess to having been darkly amused; in life, too, Richard always took his time.

As two years ticked toward three, though, I began to wonder. Had Richard been forgotten in a fridge somewhere? Near the third anniversary of his death, I called to inquire. The administrator cheerfully informed me that Richard had just "completed the program"—akin to graduating, I suppose. She offered to mail his cremated remains. I agreed but then realized I needed to drive him home myself, as a ritual of completing our circle.

So, on a warm afternoon in early December, I set off on the familiar trip to Denver. As the highway wound up Trout Creek Pass, I experienced a kind of temporal confusion that had become familiar, if no less disconcerting. Time slid across itself: It seemed as if Richard had just died, and, simultaneously, our years together felt like a dream barely related to the now.

That confusion comes partly from grief and partly from the profound changes we make in accommodating loss. In his poem "Spoken For," Li-Young Lee calls death a "rock" propping open the window of life "to admit the jasmine." Richard's death certainly threw wide the window of my life. Losing my other half forced me to stretch in ways I would not have chosen but that have enriched my self-confidence and my understanding of what I offer to life.

My biggest challenge was, frankly, money: Brain-cancer bills threatened to swallow my only real asset, the property containing the house and his studio. I needed to sell it to raise cash, but both buildings were unfinished. Nor could I afford to hire out that work. That left me one option: do it myself. I had never even turned on any of Richard's impressive array of power tools and machines, much less used them. No matter. Friends patiently taught me how to hang doors, trim windows and cabinets, mill boards, and cut sheet metal and stone. To my great surprise, I discovered my inner "tool girl": I loved the work, the equipment and materials, and the sense of competence using both gave me. When the big house and shop were finished, I helped design and build a small, passive-solar house for myself and eventually went on to renovate several other houses.

On my way to Denver that afternoon, I passed familiar landmarks: the exit we would have taken to visit Mom and Dad, the parkway where Richard and I had walked when we'd learned of his second set of tumors, the Starbucks that had been my refuge whenever he was in the hospital, and the VA hospital itself. On the CU medical school campus, I drove past Fisher House, where we had lived for that winter of radiation, and on to the anatomy lab, where I would retrieve his remains.

At the administrator's office, I mentioned that I planned to stop at Richard's favorite spots on the way home and take photos, documenting our final journey. The administrator suggested starting with the new memorial garden outside the building.

I placed the box of Richard on the garden wall—what was left of him was surprisingly hefty, weighing nearly ten pounds—and snapped a photo. And then chuckled through tears when I recognized *Corpus Callosum*, the sculpture he had admired, photobombing the background. Then I carried the box to Red, the Toyota truck I now drove, and settled Richard in the passenger seat next to the split-ash picnic basket we had used on every road trip.

Next stop was the "wave rock," a boulder Richard had lusted after alongside the highway into the foothills. Each time we had passed the sinuous, ton-size rock, Richard had mulled over how to retrieve it for a sculpture he imagined. I posed the box, told him where we were, shot a photo, wiped my eyes, returned with him to the truck, and drove on.

I stopped again at the coffee shop in the mountains where we always filled our to-go cups, and giggled at the absurdity of buying a cup of Richard's favorite dark-roast coffee for his remains. I did anyway.

Next was a cliff on the way up Kenosha Pass where Richard had picked up the boulder he had carved into a sink for the guest cottage. And then the viewpoint atop the pass where we always stopped to gaze across South Park at the peaks visible from our house. "Let's go there," he would say with a grin, pointing at the far horizon. And we did. Now I did, alone.

The sun had set by the time we reached home. As I carried the box of Richard into my small house, I heard a warbling song: the house-finch melody Richard used to whistle to Molly. A house finch singing in December? Or Richard's spirit. Whichever—the song brought a smile.

Inside, I carefully poured the gritty remains into a porcelain jar crafted by an artist whose work Richard had admired at the Salida gallery that sold his sculptures. I placed the jar, with its silk-smooth, flame-swirled surface, on a built-in shelf made of flagstones left over from the patio we had laid together. Then I added the foil chocolate wrapper that said, *Love every moment.*

Richard and I did not love every moment. We were not perfect. But we did do our best to embrace what life gave us, and to share those gifts. To live with love—not just romantic love but the genuine attachment we humans feel for each other, for other species, and for this living world as a whole. I think that kind of love is the greatest gift we have to offer. Love asks us to lead with our hearts, to accept flaws and hardships and failures as openly as joys and triumphs, and to be as true to ourselves as we can. Love is that rare blessing that increases when shared. Opening ourselves to feeling the love around us, even in our endings, fills our spirits, calms our restless searching, quiets our yearning for more: more money, more possessions, more success, more power. When we accept that all-embracing love, whatever we have in life is truly enough.

That time of journeying with dying—both Mom's and Richard's—taught me that death is not to be feared. It is not pretty, or easy, or simple, but death is an integral part of being human—and, paradoxically, of being alive. We enrich our living by making peace with it and by doing our best to go through the passage mindfully and with as much grace as possible. By walking our endings in the light of what we love, not what we fear. By learning to love life generously enough to, in Rilke's words, include life's "other half" in our love.

Another thing I learned is that grief is in part the measure of our love. The greater the love, the stronger and longer our journey with grief. Time wears away the sharpest edge of loss, but grief is a trickster, surprising us at unexpected times and in unexpected forms. Grief is a process, not something you can postpone or "get over"; you can't rush through, skip, or bypass it. You live with it and eventually live beyond it, riding the currents of life.

I'm not saying embracing death is easy. No transition so momentous and consequential is ever easy. Nor should it be. But it offers essential wisdom about living.

Walking mindfully with those who are dying teaches us who we are and what matters most. It offers us an opportunity to leave our baggage behind and to forgive—ourselves and others. The practice of accepting our losses, of accepting that there is nothing that needs to—or can—be done, offers us the opportunity to listen and simply be. To judge less and learn more.

The person I am was shaped both by loving and by losing—by the yin and the yang. We who witness the journey around that final arc of our cycle are indelibly changed, our hearts cracked open and our lives re-formed by the reality that nothing lasts. All is impermanent—except love. The truth is, love is what sustains us, always.

Hence this story, which I offer as a ray of light and a reminder that love lives, thrives, and surprises us throughout life, even when we feel most despairing of our future and that of this world. We can choose to lead with our hearts and dance our best steps along the way—hard as it may be—buoyed by the knowledge that life persists, new green sprouting from the ashes, poppies blooming, condors soaring the skies again. To be truly alive, our days fluttering like prayer flags of gratitude, hearts open to the knowledge that when the time comes, we will cycle on, our atoms dancing in life's eternal circle. The one where any end is also a beginning.

*your heartbeat echoes*
*steady as condor wingbeats*
*riding the wind home*

# a c k n o w l e d g m e n t s

So many people helped along the way. Thank you all for your kindness, patience, and wisdom; for listening and laughing; for offering a helping hand or walking alongside us. For caring.

Special thanks to the medical professionals involved with Richard's care, including Dr. Mary Reeves; Dr. Adams and the ER staff at Salida Memorial Hospital ER; the staff at the Salida Veterans Affairs clinic; and the staff and volunteers at Angel of Shavano Hospice in Salida, especially hospice nurse Will Archuletta and aide Helen Betancourt.

From our stints at the VA hospital in Denver, thanks especially to Dr. Sarah Kuykendall, Dr. Brooke Allen, and Dr. Filley in Neurology; medical student Dave Otten; Dr. Brega, Dr. Ho, and Nurse Practitioner Fran in Neurosurgery; in Oncology, Dr. Catherine Klein; Natalie DeVille, Social Work; in Palliative Care, psychologist Elizabeth Holman and Sarah Osani, Social Work; all of the nurses in both ICUs who took such good care of Richard; and Phil in Occupational Therapy. And at the UC Health Anschutz Cancer Pavillion, Dr. Chen and the staff of the radiation clinic.

For Mom's care, deep gratitude to the staff of Denver Visiting Nurses, especially nurses Callie and Pam and hospice aide Sharon. Also wonderful Monica, Mom's nonmedical aide.

Thanks, too, to the staff at the Denver Fisher House for making us so comfortable, and to Mayli Perkins and the staff at the Starbucks at Sixth and Colorado for cheering us on.

Gratitude as well to bodywork practitioners Nicky Leach of Santa Fe, and Denise Ackert and Jeannie Peters of Salida.

Thank you to the entire Salida community, who came together to support us so generously, especially Kerry and Dave Nelson, Maggie and Tony Niemann, Beverly Gray, Roberta Smith, Kathie Younghans, Mark and Brenda Wiard, Doris and Bill LeRoy, Lisa Marvel, Jeff Donlan and Laura Hendrie, Jerry Scavezze and Susan Bethany, Toni Tischer, Geraldine Alexander, CC Barton, Nicole and Harry Hansen, Marilyn Whitney, Cathy and the late Kent Haruf, Sherrie York, Annie Jacob, Ellen and Don Bauder, Katie and Bob Grether, Kathie and the late Steve Stucko, Bob Spencer, Jeff Schweitzer and Margie Sohl, and the Strawns: B, the late Mel, and Ben.

A huge thank you to the community of my blog readers, who gave us so much encouragement and support.

Special gratitude to friends Susan Kask, Tom Huizenga and Valeska Hilbig, Dave and Nancy Mayer, Grant Pound, Tim and Leanna Boers, Betsy and Geoff Blakeslee, Terry Carwile, Blanche Sobottke, Ann Vileisis and Tim Palmer, Laura and Sarah Arnow, Dale Doremus, Julie Weston and Gerry Morrison, Terry and Steve McLellan, Dave and Jan Lee, Jim Bittel, Louella Pizzuti, Jay and Connie Moody, Judy Siddle, Peg Logan, Rolfe Larson, and Mariela.

Thank you to my many writing friends and colleagues, especially my amazing agent, Elizabeth Trupin-Pulli. Also to Susan Wittig Albert, the late Debra Winegarten, the late Barry Lopez, Nancy Fay, Page Lambert, Theresa May, Penny Harter, Priscilla Stuckey, Jane Kirkpatrick, Jenny Barry, Craig Childs, Steve Trimble, Helen Thorpe, Kathleen Dean Moore, Parker Huber and the Crestone nature writers, the members of the Story Circle Network WIP group, Colorado Authors' League, Wyoming Writers, and the members of Women Writing the West. And to the Literary Ladies of Santa Fe—Anne Hillerman, Jean Schaumberg, Elizabeth

Trupin-Pulli, Dawn Wink, Lucy Moore, Karima Alavi, and Lesley Poling-Kempes—whose friendship and encouragement nurture me. To Brooke Warner, publisher of She Writes Press, for her belief in women's voices and stories, and to editorial managers Lauren Wise and Shannon Green, astute copy editor Annie Tucker, and Julie Metz, for the gorgeous cover design.

Deepest gratitude also to Jordan Young and the Women's International Study Center in Santa Fe for the generous writing residency, and to casita mates DS Magid and Stanlie James. And to the Mesa Refuge in California, and my suite mate Alia Malek, walking companion extraordinaire. Also to Connie Holsinger and the Terra Foundation, and Grant Pound and Colorado Art Ranch for writing and residency time.

Thank you to the extended Cabe clan for the gift of Richard and Molly in my life. Special thanks to Andrew Cabe, who shared such a close bond with his Unc and who helped build the big house and helped finish it. And to Jennifer Cabe, for wisdom, love, and support.

To my family: Molly Cabe, daughter of my heart; my dad and mom, the late Bob and Joan Tweit; my brother, Bill Tweit, and his wife, Lucy Winter; and my three nieces, Alice Winter Tweit, Sienna Bryant, and Heather Roland, and their families. I love you! You provided the circle of love that we needed.

Last but certainly not least, thank you to DeWitt, who walked into my life after this journey—an unimagined blessing.

# about the author

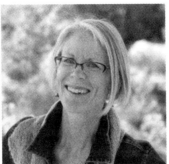

credit: Robert Muller

SUSAN J. TWEIT is a plant biologist who began her career working in the wilderness studying wildfires, grizzly bear habitat and sagebrush ecosystems. She turned to writing when she realized she loved telling the stories in the data. She is an award-winning author of twelve books, including a previous memoir, *Walking Nature Home*, and has been published in magazines and newspapers including *Audubon*, *Popular Mechanics*, the *Denver Post*, and the *Los Angeles Times*. Her essays and commentaries have been collected in numerous anthologies, and heard on regional public radio. She is co-founder of the Border Book Festival and Audubon Rockies' Be A Habitat Hero Project, and an active member of Women Writing the West and Story Circle Network. Visit her online at www.susanjtweit.com. Tweit, a Quaker, writes from the high desert outside Santa Fe, New Mexico, where deer and coyotes saunter through her garden and stars stud a dark night sky.